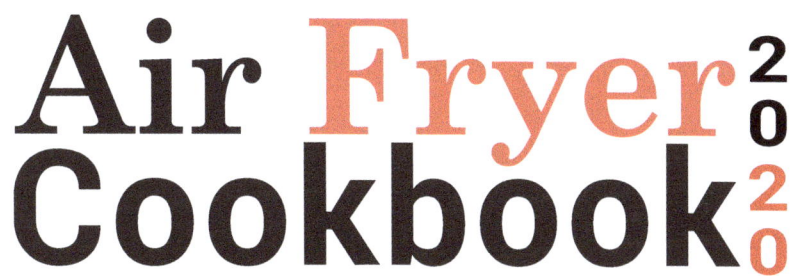

The 600 Deliciously Simple Recipes For Your Air Fryer

Text Copyright © Gina Newman

All rights reserved. No part of this guide may be reproduced in any form without permission in writing from the publisher except in the case of brief quotations embodied in critical articles or reviews.

Legal & Disclaimer

The information contained in this book and its contents is not designed to replace or take the place of any form of medical or professional advice; and is not meant to replace the need for independent medical, financial, legal or other professional advice or services, as may be required. The content and information in this book has been provided for educational and entertainment purposes only.

The content and information contained in this book has been compiled from sources deemed reliable, and it is accurate to the best of the Author's knowledge, information and belief. However, the Author cannot guarantee its accuracy and validity and cannot be held liable for any errors and/or omissions. Further, changes are periodically made to this book as and when needed. Where appropriate and/or necessary, you must consult a professional (including but not limited to your doctor, attorney, financial advisor or such other professional advisor) before using any of the suggested remedies, techniques, or information in this book.

Upon using the contents and information contained in this book, you agree to hold harmless the Author from and against any damages, costs, and expenses, including any legal fees potentially resulting from the application of any of the information provided by this book. This disclaimer applies to any loss, damages or injury caused by the use and application, whether directly or indirectly, of any advice or information presented, whether for breach of contract, tort, negligence, personal injury, criminal intent, or under any other cause of action.

You agree to accept all risks of using the information presented inside this book.

You agree that by continuing to read this book, where appropriate and/or necessary, you shall consult a professional (including but not limited to your doctor, attorney, or financial advisor or such other advisor as needed) before using any of the suggested remedies, techniques, or information in this book.

Contents

Introduction 1

    Chapter One **Introducing the Air Fryer 2**

    Chapter Two **Breakfast Recipes 9**

    Chapter Three **Lunch Recipes 27**

    Chapter Four **Snacks Recipes 128**

    Chapter Five **Dinner Recipes 158**

    Chapter Six **Dessert Recipes 173**

Conclusion 197

Introduction

Currently, cooking is not something as heavy as it was thanks to the use of many electrical appliances. Buying any appliance requires knowing how the different models work and what they all do. The Air Fryer is one household appliance that is most present in our kitchens. However, times have changed and today we care more about our health and nutrition. For this reason, we have reduced our consumption of fatty foods in recent years. Oil-free fryers have become a success.

But how can a deep fryer cook without oil? In practice, these appliances are small ovens that provide high-speed air convection cooking. Thanks to this, you can get crispy foods without the need for oil, or by adding just a little.

In the market, you have at your disposal countless models. When choosing your fryer without oil, what you have to take into account is the number of diners you usually cook for, the free space you have in your kitchen, and the functions you would like to enjoy.

If you want to buy an air fryer but you don't know which one, this book will surely help you choose the one that best suits your needs. You will also find how to prepare 200 healthy recipes.

Enjoy it!

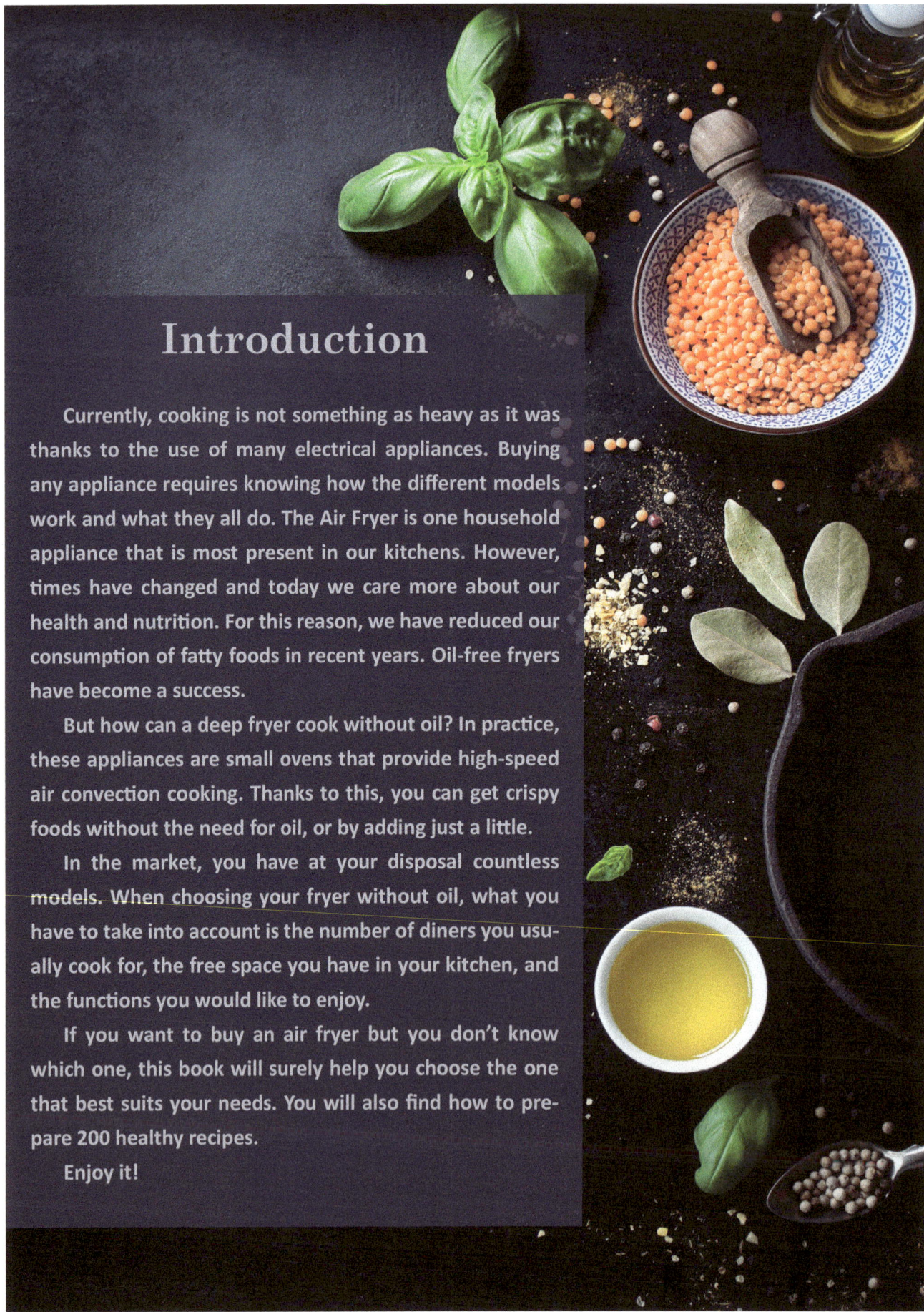

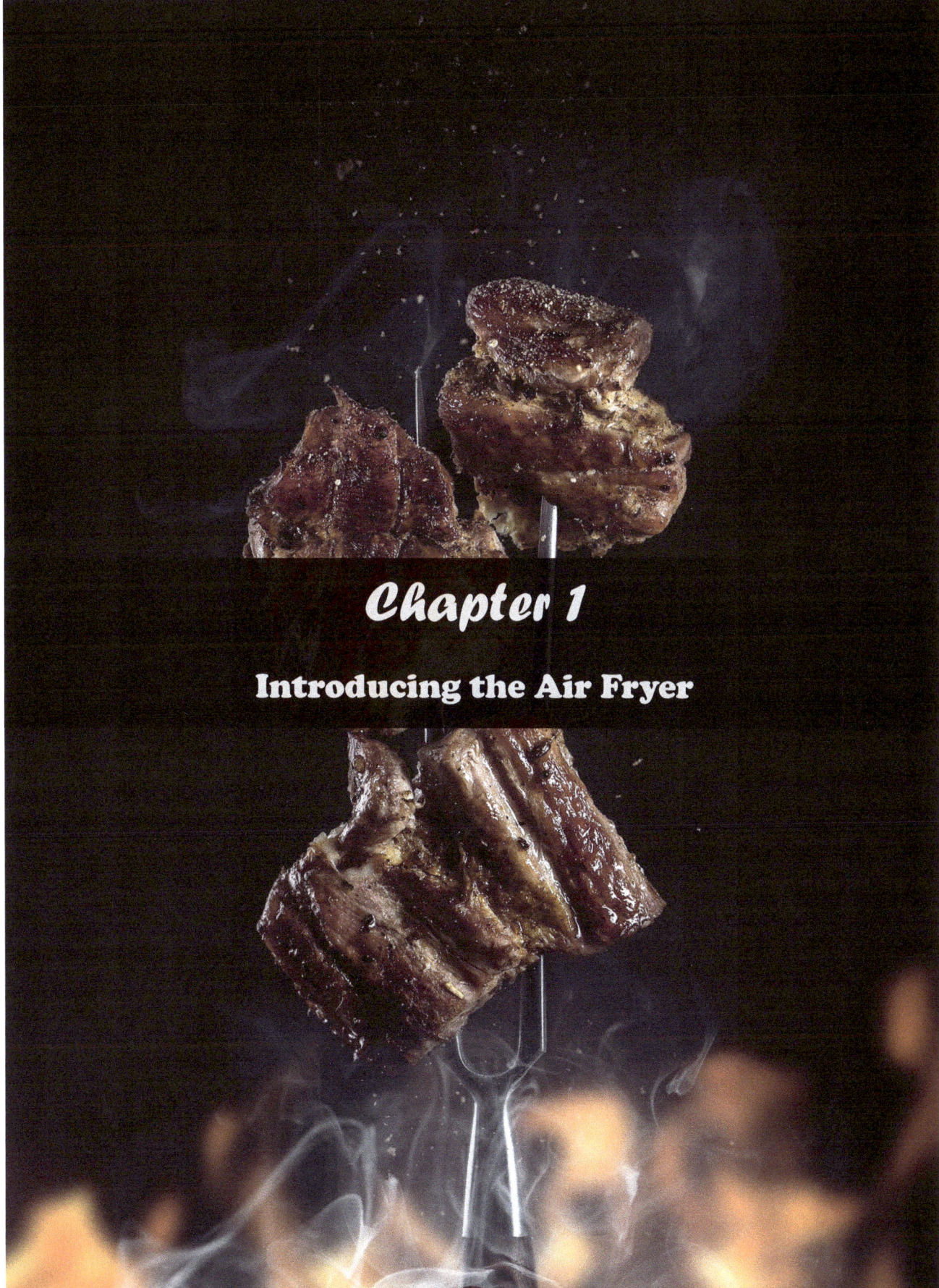

Chapter 1

Introducing the Air Fryer

Since air fryers appeared, there has been a lot of speculation about their use and guarantees, so the first thing we are going to clarify to our readers is: what is an air fryer?

It is an appliance that mainly uses a hot air system, which is distributed through some fans, to cook food - this is how the air fryer works, although this depends on the model and may vary slightly.

When you use an air fryer, you have a lot of benefits. They are easy to use and clean, they do not cause odors because the air or steam they expel is infinitely less than that of conventional fryers, and of course the lower consumption of fats and cholesterol in the food is a highlight. Food is cooked with up to 80% less oil.

How does an air fryer work?

Fryers use Rapid Air technology to cook any type of food that would otherwise submerge it in fat. This new technology works by circulating air at high degrees, up to 200°C, to "fry" foods like fish, deep fryers, 21 chips, cakes, chicken, and more. Rapid Air technology is bringing a new era of kitchen appliances and a new generation of cooking methods together. Air fryers deliver perfectly better crisp, golden Taurus fryers with less fat, compared to traditional cooking methods.

The benefits of air fryer

Avoid excess oil

When you remove the food from a pan with oil, it often has a very marked oil flavor. To avoid this, nutritionists recommend frying food in a deep fryer without oil. This is recommended because fried food is usually cooked in plenty of hot oil. The oil-free fryer eradicates the flavor variable.

You do not have to worry about the temperature

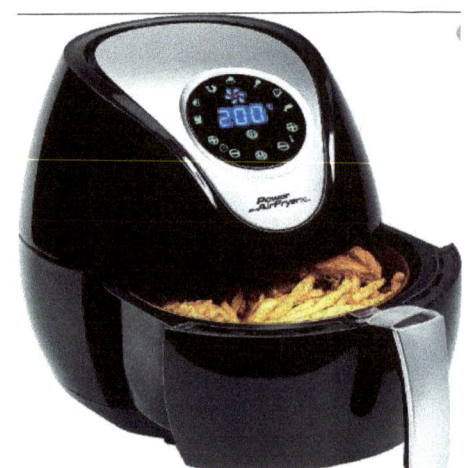

If you are a regular cook you will know that not all ingredients are fried at the same temperature. The fryer takes care of it. These artifacts incorporate a heat regulator. They give you temperatures for meats, vegetables, and dough, so you no longer have to buy those expensive thermometers. Making sure your food is perfectly fried is easier.

Include timer

Manufacturers have created some timer fryer designs. These indicate, through a sound or light, that the food may be extracted. Those that do not have this function have the time specified along with the temperature corresponding to each ingredient.

Easy to use with a computerized system

Using an oil-free deep fryer does not require professional culinary skills. They have a digital control panel that takes care of all the settings. They also add the advantage of speed and working time over oil-free fryers. They are almost automatic in operation.

They have a considerable capacity

They come in sizes with a capacity for at least two or three dishes, which means that you can cook several portions simultaneously. In this way, it will take little time to satisfy your diners.

Save oil by not needing it

If you fry your food in a common frying pan, you will have to keep adding oil to the frying pan repeatedly. When you use an oil-free deep fryer, food will cook in less time. It will form a film that prevents grease from seeping in. Fat and cholesterol, will no longer be a concern to your diet when you remove oil from food.

It should not be cleaned every day

Cleaning the oil from the pan where we fry food can be a very cumbersome job. Fat does not dissolve easily. With the fryer, you will not have to face this daily inconvenience. It will be enough to clean it once a week if you use it frequently.

Don't get dirty from the oil

Without the oil, there is no need to recycle or replace anything.. Its action by heat, air, and electricity makes frying healthier, faster, cleaner, and more comfortable. You will not end up with oil splashes on you or your clothing.

The operation is easily graduated

The oil-free fryer operates in the same way as a microwave or oven; you configure the minutes you want it to cook for, and the intensity. The work is autonomous. There is nothing to supervise.

Choosing your Air Fryer

If you have decided on a traditional fryer with an oil container, you must take into account three fundamental aspects: capacity, temperature range, and ease of cleaning.

• Fryer capacity:

Will depend on the number of people you usually cook for. For example, for 1.2 kilos of food, you need a 3-liter oil fryer.

• The temperature range:

Although it is not recommended to fry at a very high temperature, it is interesting that you can fry at a low temperature for the most delicate foods, such as fish.

- *Cleanliness:*

Nothing is more unpleasant than a dirty deep fryer. They are available with an oil filter, to keep them clean for longer. Also, it must be removable, in this way it is easier to clean it, even put it in the dishwasher.

5 Tips for Air Frying

Tip #1: Dry the food well

Before air frying, dry anything (without breading) that you want crispy or golden, such as meat, fish, and vegetables.

Tip #2: Avoid overfilling the basket

An air fryer relies on a fan to circulate hot air and cook food quickly. If you fill the basket, this prevents hot air from reaching all of the food, which slows the cooking down and can give uneven results. Some models have lines for maximum fill, and the manual can also provide full if the basket does not have a maximum fill line.

Tip #3: Check food frequently

Unlike cooking food in the oven, you cannot turn on the light and check the cooking of food through the window. With an air fryer you can't see ingredients as they cook, as they are placed in a drawer-style basket, making it more difficult to get an idea of how it is going. To avoid overcooked food, check it from time to time while cooking. (On some models, this is as simple as pulling out the drawer, but on others, you may need to stop cooking before doing so; specific information can be found in your manual.)

Tip #4: Flip the food over while cooking

Use tongs or shake the basket during cooking for more uniform results.

Tip #5: Experiment with home favorites

Sure, store-bought potato chips taste great, but an air fryer makes the job easier. For homemade crispy potato chips, cut potatoes into even pieces and soak them in water for 30 minutes. Then drain, rinse, dry, and lightly coat with oil before air frying.

Measurement Conversions: *Mass units' conversion table*

	Kilogram (kg)	Atomic Unit of mass (u)	Slug	Ounce (oz.)	Pound (lb.)
1 Kilogram	1	$6.022*10^{26}$	$6.852*10^{-2}$	35.27	2.205
1 Atomic Unit of Mass	$1.661*10^{-27}$	1	$1.138*10^{-28}$	$5.857*10^{-27}$	$3.661*10^{-27}$
1 Slug	14.59	$8.788*10^{27}$	1	514.8	32.17
1 ounce	$2.835*10^{-2}$	$1.707*10^{25}$	$1.943*10^{-3}$	1	$6.250*10^{-2}$
1 Pound	0.4536	$2.732*10^{26}$	$3.108*10^{-2}$	16	1
1 Ton	$9.072*10^{2}$	$5.463*10^{29}$	62.16	$3.200*10^{4}$	2000

Gina Newman

Volume Units Conversion Table

	Multiply by / Convert to							
Convert from	cubic metre	cubic decimetre	cubic centimetre	cubic millimetre	hectoliters	liters	centiliters	milliliters
cubic meters	1	10^3	10^6	10^9	10	10^3	10^5	10^6
cubic decimeters	10^{-3}	1	10^3	10^6	0.01	1	100	10^3
cubic centimeters	10^{-6}	10^{-3}	1	10^3	10^{-5}	10^{-3}	0.1	1
cubic millimeters	10^{-9}	10^{-6}	10^{-3}	1	10^{-8}	10^{-6}	10^{-4}	10^{-3}
hectoliters	0.1	10^2	10^5	10^8	1	10^2	10^4	10^5
liters	10^{-3}	1	10^3	10^6	10^{-2}	1	10^2	10^3
centiliters	10^{-4}	10^{-2}	10	10^4	10^{-4}	10^{-2}	1	10
milliliters	10^{-6}	10^{-3}	1	10^3	10^{-5}	10^{-3}	0.1	1
cubic inches	1.6×10^{-5}	1.6×10^{-2}	16.4	1.64×10^4	1.64×10^{-4}	1.64×10^{-2}	1.64	16.4
cubic feet	2.8×10^{-2}	28.3	2.83×10^4	2.83×10^7	0.28	28.3	2.83×10^3	2.83×10^4
cubic yards	0.765	765	7.65×10^5	7.65×10^8	7.65	765	7.65×10^4	7.65×10^5
us liquid gallons	3.79×10^{-3}	3.79	3.79×10^3	3.79×10^6	3.79×10^{-2}	3.79	379	3.79×10^3
us dry gallons	4.4×10^{-3}	4.4	4.4×10^3	4.4×10^6	4.4×10^{-2}	4.4	440	4.4×10^3
imp liquid gallons	4.55×10^{-3}	4.55	4.55×10^3	4.55×10^6	4.56×10^{-2}	4.55	455	4.55×10^3
barrels (oil)	0.16	159	1.59×10^5	1.59×10^8	1.59	159	1.59×10^4	1.59×10^5
cups	2.4×10^{-4}	0.24	236.6	2.37×10^5	2.37×10^{-3}	0.236	23.7	236.6
fluid ounces (UK)	2.8×10^{-5}	2.8×10^{-2}	28.4	2.8×10^4	2.8×10^{-4}	2.8×10^{-2}	2.84	28.4
fluid ounces (US)	2.96×10^{-5}	2.96×10^{-2}	29.6	2.96×10^4	2.96×10^{-4}	2.96×10^{-2}	2.96	29.6
pints (UK)	5.68×10^{-4}	0.568	568	5.68×10^5	5.68×10^{-3}	0.568	56.8	568

Volume Units Conversion Table:

Convert from	Multiply by — Convert to										
	cubic inches	cubic feet	cubic yards	us liquid gallons	us dry gallons	imp liquid gallons	barrels (oil)	cups	fluid ounces (UK)	fluid ounces (US)	pints (UK)
cubic metre	$6.1 \cdot 10^4$	35.3	1.308	264.2	227	220	6.29	4227	$3.52 \cdot 10^4$	$3.38 \cdot 10^4$	1760
cubic decimetre	61.02	0.035	$1.3 \cdot 10^{-3}$	0.264	0.227	0.22	0.006	4.23	35.2	33.8	1.76
cubic centimetre	0.061	$3.5 \cdot 10^{-5}$	$1.3 \cdot 10^{-6}$	$2.64 \cdot 10^{-4}$	$2.27 \cdot 10^{-4}$	$2.2 \cdot 10^{-4}$	$6.29 \cdot 10^{-6}$	$4.2 \cdot 10^{-3}$	$3.5 \cdot 10^{-2}$	$3.34 \cdot 10^{-2}$	$1.76 \cdot 10^{-3}$
cubic millimetre	$6.1 \cdot 10^{-5}$	$3.5 \cdot 10^{-8}$	$1.31 \cdot 10^{-9}$	$2.64 \cdot 10^{-7}$	$2.27 \cdot 10^{-7}$	$2.2 \cdot 10^{-7}$	$6.3 \cdot 10^{-9}$	$4.2 \cdot 10^{-6}$	$3.5 \cdot 10^{-5}$	$3.4 \cdot 10^{-5}$	$1.76 \cdot 10^{-6}$
hectoliters	$6.1 \cdot 10^3$	3.53	0.13	26.4	22.7	22	0.63	423	$3.5 \cdot 10^3$	3381	176
liters	61	$3.5 \cdot 10^{-2}$	$1.3 \cdot 10^{-3}$	0.26	0.23	0.22	$6.3 \cdot 10^{-3}$	4.2	35.2	33.8	1.76
centiliters	0.61	$3.5 \cdot 10^{-4}$	$1.3 \cdot 10^{-5}$	$2.6 \cdot 10^{-3}$	$2.3 \cdot 10^{-3}$	$2.2 \cdot 10^{-3}$	$6.3 \cdot 10^{-5}$	$4.2 \cdot 10^{-2}$	0.35	0.338	$1.76 \cdot 10^{-2}$
milliliters	$6.1 \cdot 10^{-2}$	$3.5 \cdot 10^{-5}$	$1.3 \cdot 10^{-6}$	$2.6 \cdot 10^{-4}$	$2.3 \cdot 10^{-4}$	$2.2 \cdot 10^{-4}$	$6.3 \cdot 10^{-6}$	$4.2 \cdot 10^{-3}$	$3.5 \cdot 10^{-2}$	$3.4 \cdot 10^{-2}$	$1.76 \cdot 10^{-3}$
cubic inches	1	$5.79 \cdot 10^{-4}$	$2.1 \cdot 10^{-5}$	$4.3 \cdot 10^{-3}$	$3.7 \cdot 10^{-3}$	$3.6 \cdot 10^{-3}$	10^{-4}	$6.9 \cdot 10^{-2}$	0.58	0.55	$2.9 \cdot 10^{-2}$
cubic feet	1728	1	0.037	7.48	6.43	6.23	0.18	119.7	997	958	49.8
cubic yards	$4.7 \cdot 10^4$	27	1	202	173.6	168.2	4.8	3232	$2.69 \cdot 10^4$	$2.59 \cdot 10^4$	1345
us liquid gallons	231	0.134	$4.95 \cdot 10^{-3}$	1	0.86	0.83	0.024	16	133.2	128	6.7
us dry gallons	268.8	0.156	$5.76 \cdot 10^{-3}$	1.16	1	0.97	0.028	18.62	155	148.9	7.75
imp liquid gallons	277.4	0.16	$5.9 \cdot 10^{-3}$	1.2	1.03	1	0.029	19.2	160	153.7	8
barrels (oil)	9702	5.61	0.21	42	36.1	35	1	672	5596	5376	279.8
cups	14.4	$8.4 \cdot 10^{-3}$	$3.1 \cdot 10^{-4}$	$6.2 \cdot 10^{-2}$	$5.4 \cdot 10^{-2}$	$5.2 \cdot 10^{-2}$	$1.5 \cdot 10^{-3}$	1	8.3	8	0.4
fluid ounces (UK)	1.73	10^{-3}	$3.7 \cdot 10^{-5}$	$7.5 \cdot 10^{-3}$	$6.45 \cdot 10^{-3}$	$6.25 \cdot 10^{-3}$	$1.79 \cdot 10^{-4}$	0.12	1	0.96	$5 \cdot 10^{-2}$
fluid ounces (US)	1.8	10^{-3}	$3.87 \cdot 10^{-5}$	$7.8 \cdot 10^{-3}$	$6.7 \cdot 10^{-3}$	$6.5 \cdot 10^{-3}$	$1.89 \cdot 10^{-4}$	0.13	1.04	1	0.052
pints (UK)	34.7	0.02	$7.4 \cdot 10^{-4}$	0.15	0.129	0.125	$3.57 \cdot 10^{-3}$	2.4	20	19.2	1

Source: https://www.engineeringtoolbox.com/volume-units-converter-d_1034.html

Gina Newman

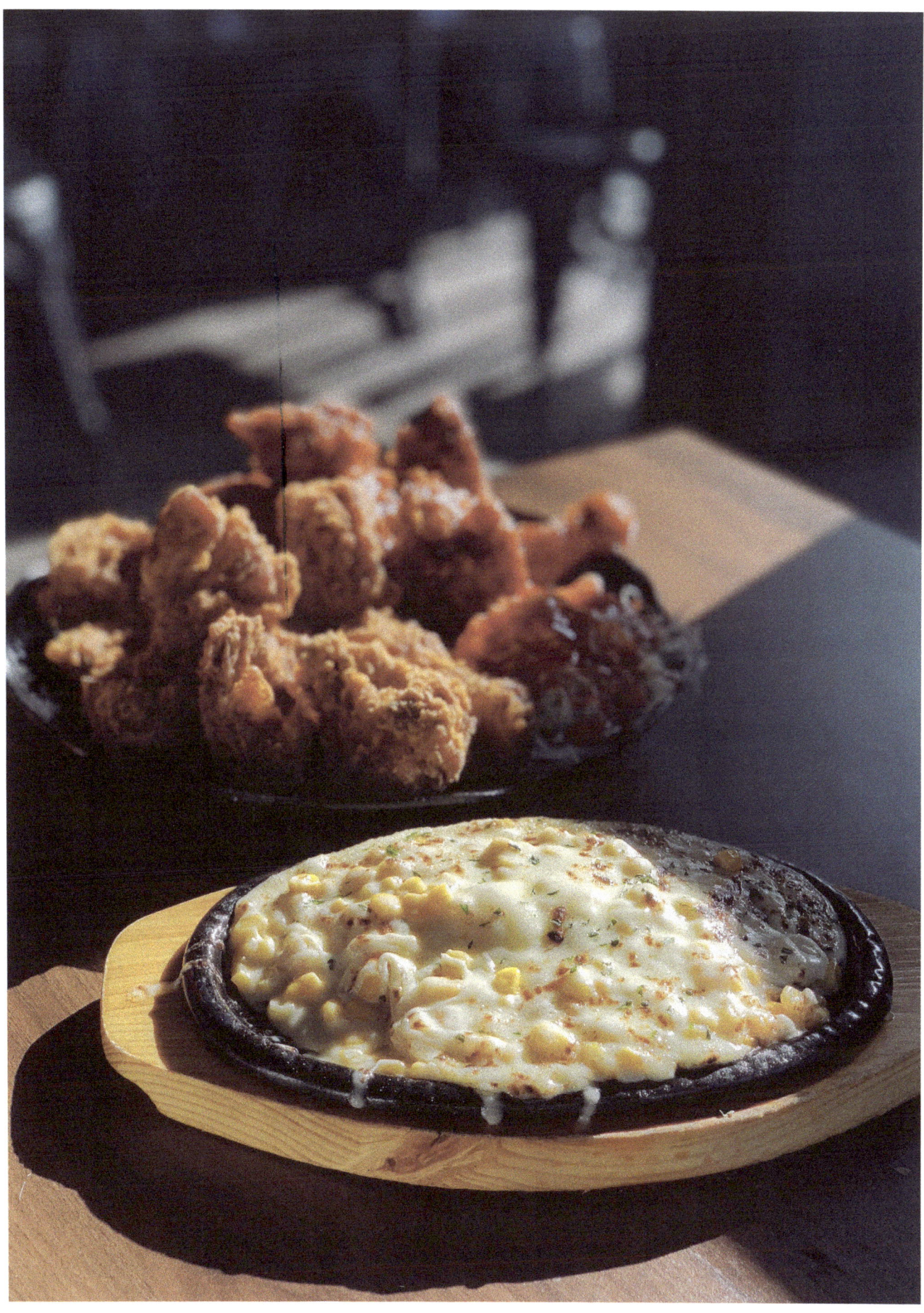

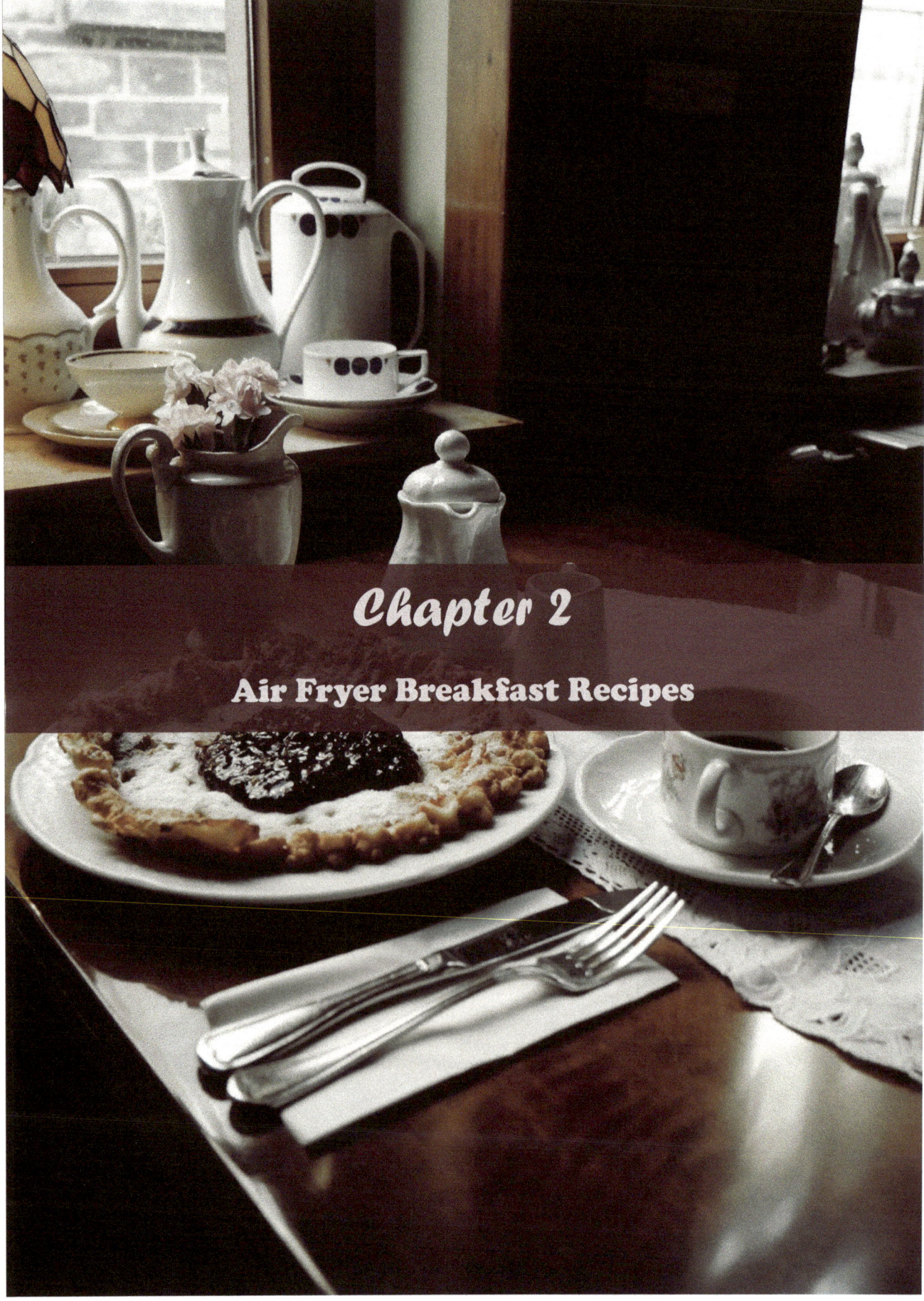

Chapter 2
Air Fryer Breakfast Recipes

FLAVORSOME

Stuffed French Toast

• Servings: 1 • Preparation time: 4 minutes • Cook time: 10 minutes •

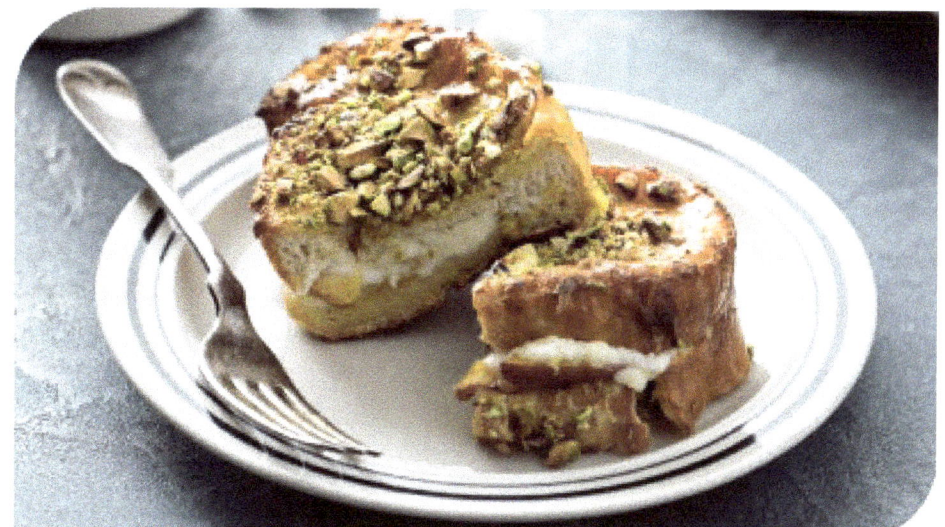

Ingredients

- 1 slice of brioche
- 4 oz. thick white cheese
- 2 eggs
- 3 tsp milk
- 6 tsp thick cream
- 1.3 oz. sugar
- ½ tsp cinnamon
- ½ tsp vanilla extract
- Cooking spray
- Crushed pistachio and maple syrup to decorate

Steps to Cook

1. Select Preheat on the Air Fryer, set to 350°F and press Start/Pause. Cut a slit in the middle of the brioche slice.

2. Fill the slit with cottage cheese. Reserve.

3. Whisk together the eggs, milk, heavy cream, sugar, cinnamon, and vanilla extract.

4. Dip the stuffed French toast in the egg mixture for 10 seconds on each side.

5. Spray each side of the French toast with the oil spray.

6. Place the French toast in the preheated air fryer and bake for 10 minutes at 350°F.

7. Carefully remove the French toast with a spatula after baking. Serve with maple syrup and crushed pistachios.

Nutritional Information

- Calories: 360
- Carbohydrates: 43g
- Fat: 12g
- Protein: 21g
- Sugar: 13g
- Cholesterol: 165mg

Streusel Coffee Muffins

• Servings: 1 • Preparation time: 2 minutes • Cook time: 10 minutes •

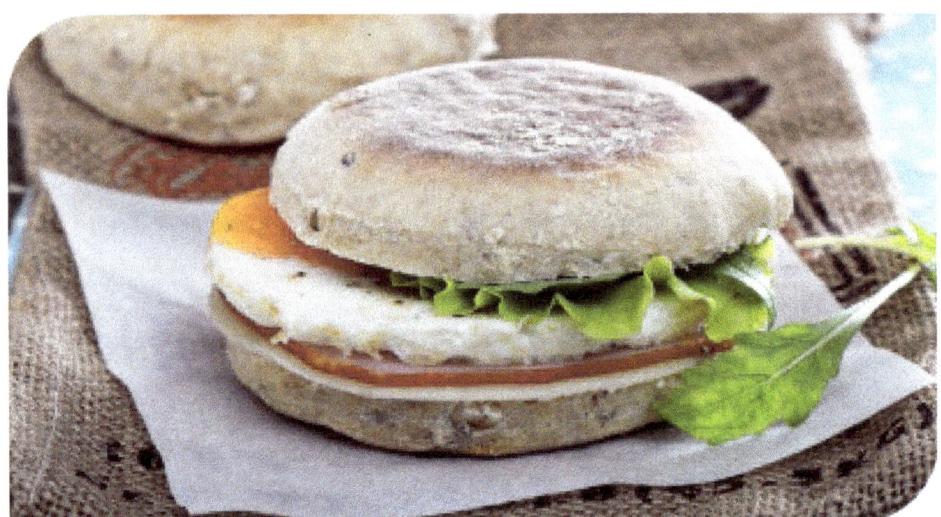

APPETIZING

Ingredients

- Cooking oil spray
- 1 slice of white cheddar cheese
- 1 slice of Canadian bacon
- 1 English muffin, cut in half
- 3 tsp hot water
- 1 large egg
- Salt and pepper

Steps to Cook

1. Drizzle the inside pan with cooking oil and place it in the air fryer.

2. Select Preheat, set to 320°F and press Start pause. Put the Canadian cheese and bacon on a half muffin.

3. Place the two halves of the muffin in the preheated air fryer. Pour the hot water and the egg into the hot pan and season with salt and pepper.

4. Select Pan, set to 10 minutes and press Start pause.

5. Take out the English muffin 7 minutes later and leave the egg for the entire duration.

6. Assemble your sandwich by placing the egg on the English muffin, then serve.

Nutritional Information

- Calories: 313.1
- Carbohydrates: 60.4g
- Fat: 7.4g
- Protein: 5.4g
- Sugar: 32.7g
- Cholesterol: 47.7mg

CRUNCHY

French Toast Sticks

• Servings: 4 • Preparation time: 5 minutes • Cook time: 10 minutes •

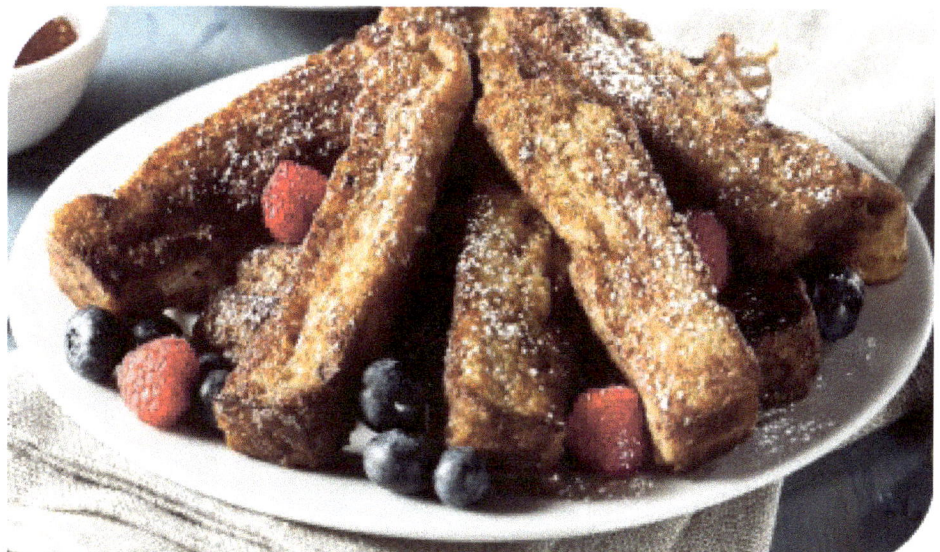

Ingredients

- 4 slices white bread,
- 2 eggs
- ¼ cup milk
- 3 tsp of maple syrup
- ½ tsp vanilla extract
- Cooking oil spray
- ½ oz. of sugar
- ½ tsp cinnamon maple syrup powder, to serve
- Powdered sugar for sprinkling

Steps to Cook

1. Cut each slice of bread into thirds to make 12 pieces. Reserve. Whisk together the eggs, milk, maple syrup, and vanilla. Select Preheat on the Air Fryer, set to 350°F and press Start/Pause. Let it warm up.

2. Dip the loaves of bread into the egg mixture and place them in the preheated air fryer. Drizzle a generous amount of cooking oil over them.

3. Bake French toast sticks for 10 minutes at 350°F. Turn the sticks halfway through cooking.

4. Mix the sugar and cinnamon in a bowl.

5. Top the French toast sticks with the cinnamon sugar mixture after cooking. Serve with maple syrup and sprinkle with sugar.

Nutritional Information

- Calories: 370.6
- Carbohydrates: 44.9g
- Fat: 19.3g
- Protein: 6.5g
- Sugar: 10.8g
- Cholesterol: 75mg

Puff pastry bites

• Servings: 9 • Preparation time: 10 minutes • Cook time: 10 minutes •

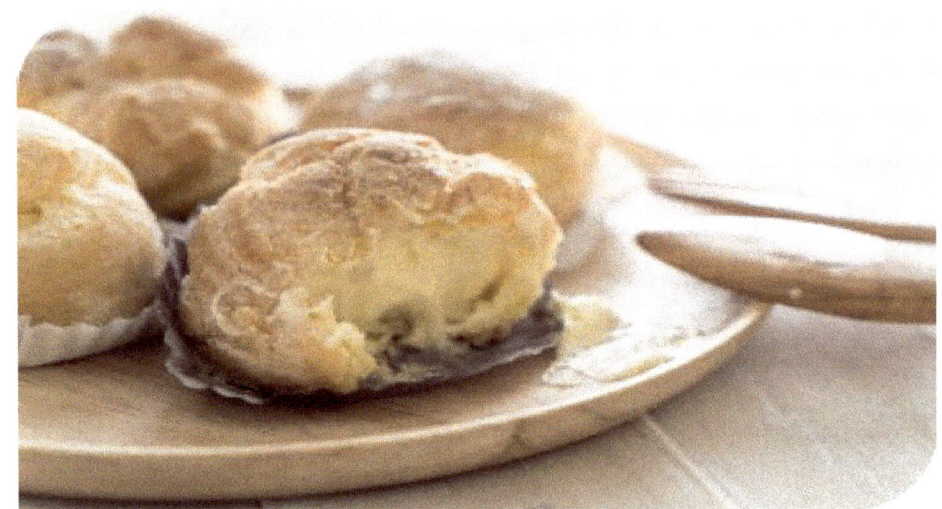

PALATABLE

Ingredients

- 7 oz. fresh or frozen puff pastry
- Topping of your choice
- 2 tbsp. milk

Steps to Cook

1. Preheat the air fryer to 400°F.

2. Cut the dough into 16 5x5 cm squares and place a level teaspoon of filling on each square.

3. Fold the dough into triangles and moisten the edges with water. Press the edges firmly with a fork.

4. Put eight triangles in the basket and brush them with milk. Lower the basket into the fryer and set the timer for 10 minutes. Remove the triangles when they are golden.

5. Cook the other triangles in the same way. Serve the triangles on a platter.

Nutritional Information

- Calories: 158
- Carbohydrates: 13g
- Fat: 11g
- Protein: 2.1g
- Sugar: 0.2g
- Cholesterol: 0mg

Tostones

• Servings: 2 • Preparation time: 2 minutes • Cook time: 8 minutes •

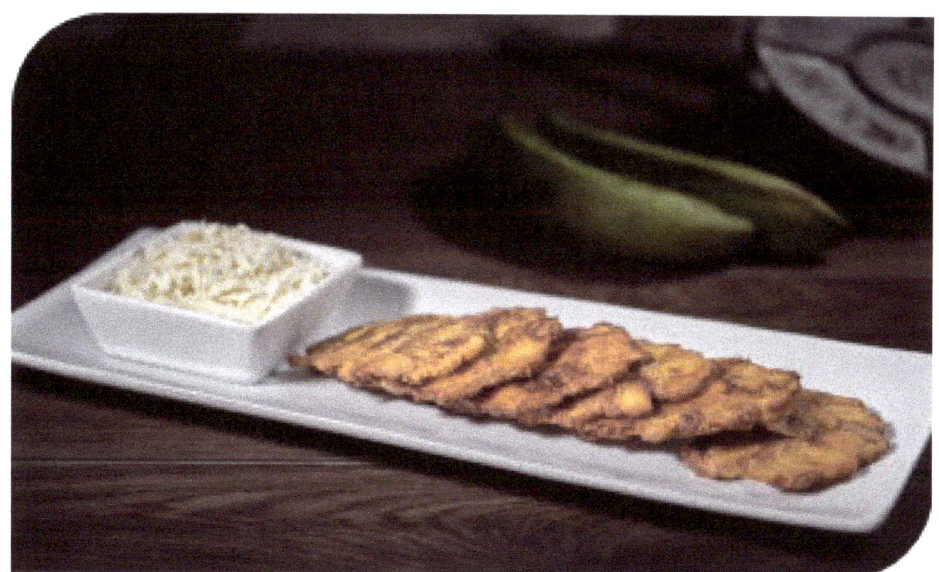

Ingredients

- 2 green bananas
- 2 tbsp. olive oil
- 1 tsp salt or more, to taste
- 1 tsp garlic powder -optional

Steps to Cook

1. Preheat the air fryer to 200ºC [400ºF].

2. Place the banana slices in the bowl of the air fryer, making sure they don't stack, and return the bowl to the air fryer.

3. Cook for 15 minutes or until light golden in color and crisp around the edges.

Nutritional Information

- Calories: 170
- Carbohydrates: 37g
- Fat: 2g
- Protein: 1g
- Sugar: 0g
- Cholesterol: 0mg

Crispy Brussels Sprouts

• Servings: 4 • Preparation time: 45 minutes • Cook time: 25 minutes •

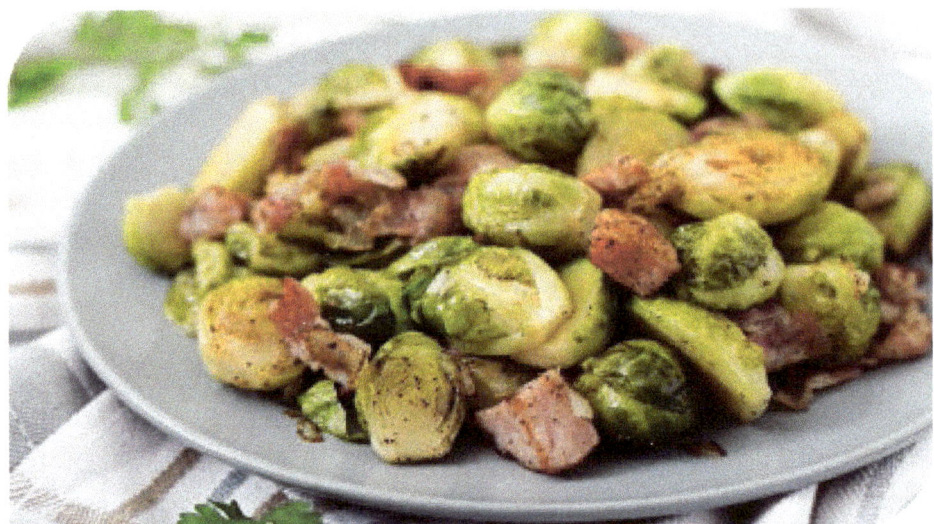

LOW FAT

Ingredients

- 1 pound Brussels sprouts, stems removed and quartered
- 2 tbsp. of oil
- Salt and pepper to taste

Steps to Cook

1. In a large bowl, mix the Brussels sprouts with the oil, salt, and pepper. Pour into the fryer basket and place in a single layer.

2. Cook in the fryer at 340° for 7 minutes. Check if the shoots are tender by poking with a fork. If they are not tender, cook at 340°F for 3 more minutes.

3. If the sprouts are tender, but not yet crisp enough, turn the air fryer to 340°F and cook for 3 minutes. Check and cook longer, if desired.

4. Season to taste.

Nutritional Information

- Calories: 56
- Carbohydrates: 11g
- Fat: 0.8g
- Protein: 4g
- Sugar: 2.7g
- Cholesterol: 0mg

Dominican Arepa

• Servings: 6 • Preparation time: 45 minutes • Cook time: 25 minutes •

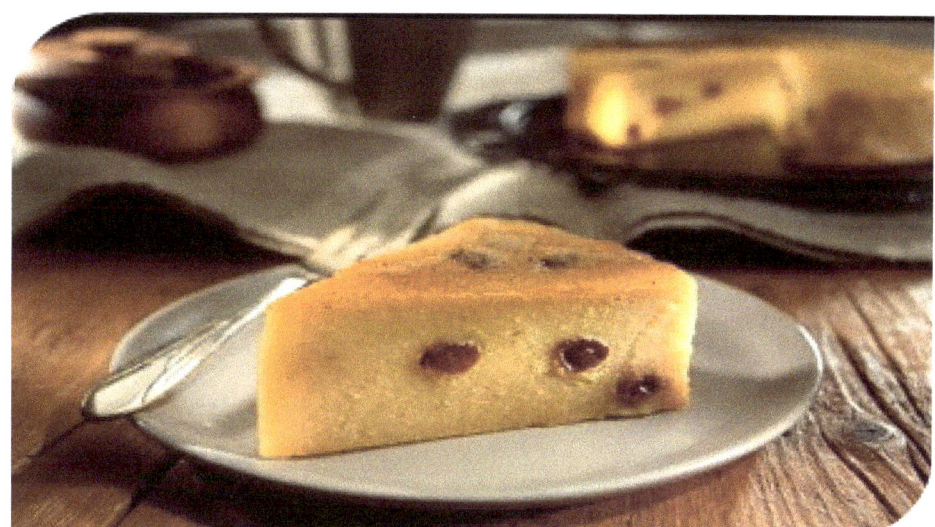

DELICIOUS

Ingredients

- 1 tbsp. of butter (to spread around the mold)
- 3 tbsp. of butter
- 2 cups cornmeal
- 3 ½ cups whole milk
- 2 ½ cups of coconut milk
- ½ tsp salt
- ½ cup raisins
- 4 cinnamon sticks
- 1 ½ cups brown sugar

Steps to Cook

1. Butter a 2 ½ liter baking pan. Heat the air fryer to 175ºC. Mix butter, cornmeal, milk, coconut milk, salt, raisins, cinnamon, and sugar. Stir the flour mixture with a spatula and pour into a pan, heating on the stove, stirring constantly to prevent sticking.

2. When mixture starts to boil, lower the temperature and continue stirring until it thickens enough that if you fill the ladle and turn it upside-down, the mixture will not fall out. Remove the cinnamon. Pour the mixture into the buttered mold and put in the air fryer basket. Bake at 170ºC for 40 minutes. Remove from oven and allow cooling to room temperature before removing from pan.

3. Serve with hot chocolate or coffee.

Nutritional Information

- Calories: 305
- Carbohydrates: 34.35g
- Fat: 16g
- Protein: 7.04g
- Sugar: 3.59g
- Cholesterol: 62mg

Air Fryer Cookbook

Cornbread

• Servings: 4 • Preparation time: 10 minutes • Cook time: 35 minutes •

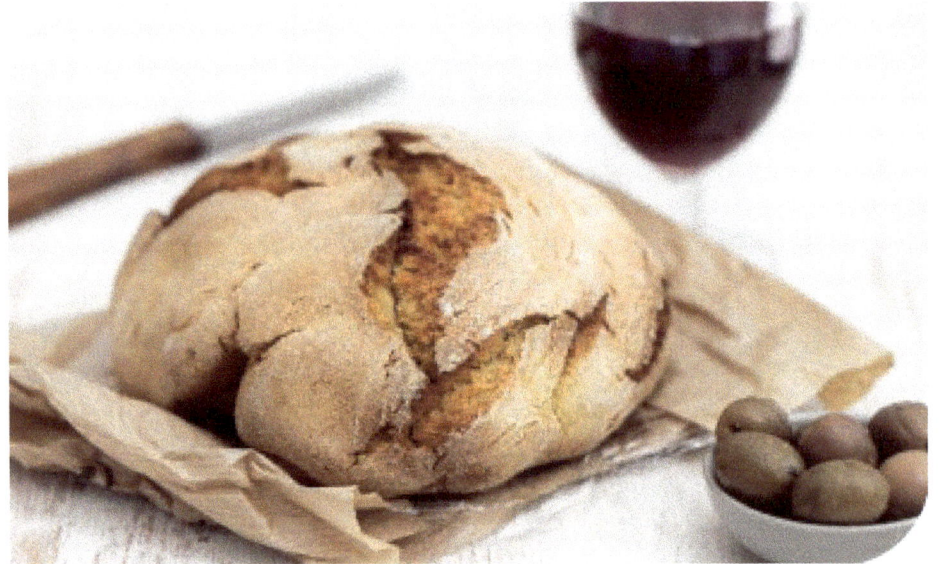

FLAVORFUL

Ingredients

Dry ingredients to mix first:

- 1 cup cornmeal
- ½ cup brown sugar
- 1 tbsp. cornstarch
- 1 tsp salt
- 1 tsp cinnamon powder

Rest of ingredients:

- 1 cup evaporated milk
- 1 tsp baking powder
- 2 medium eggs
- ½ cup butter at room temp. + extra to grease the mold
- 1/8 cup raisins (optional)

Steps to Cook

Mix dry ingredients:

1. Mix cornmeal, sugar, cornstarch, salt, and cinnamon.

2. Add the milk: pour the milk into the dry ingredients and mix. Let it sit for an hour (this is optional, but it results in a softer cornbread).

3. Grease a small nonstick pan (6-cup capacity).

Prepare the mixture:

4. Add the baking powder to the cornmeal mixture, followed by eggs and butter. Mix with a mixer until all the ingredients have been incorporated. Pour the mixture into the baking pan.

5. Put in the air fryer at 300ºF (150ºC) for 35 minutes or until you insert a toothpick and it comes out clean. Allow to cool before removing from pan.

6. Remove from the pan and serve at room temperature. Serve with hot chocolate, coffee, or a hot drink of your choice.

Nutritional Information

- Calories: 73
- Carbohydrates: 12.9g
- Fat: 1.4g
- Protein: 2.5g
- Sugar: 2.7g
- Cholesterol: 13.6mg

Broken Eggs

• Servings: 4 • Preparation time: 45 minutes • Cook time: 25 minutes •

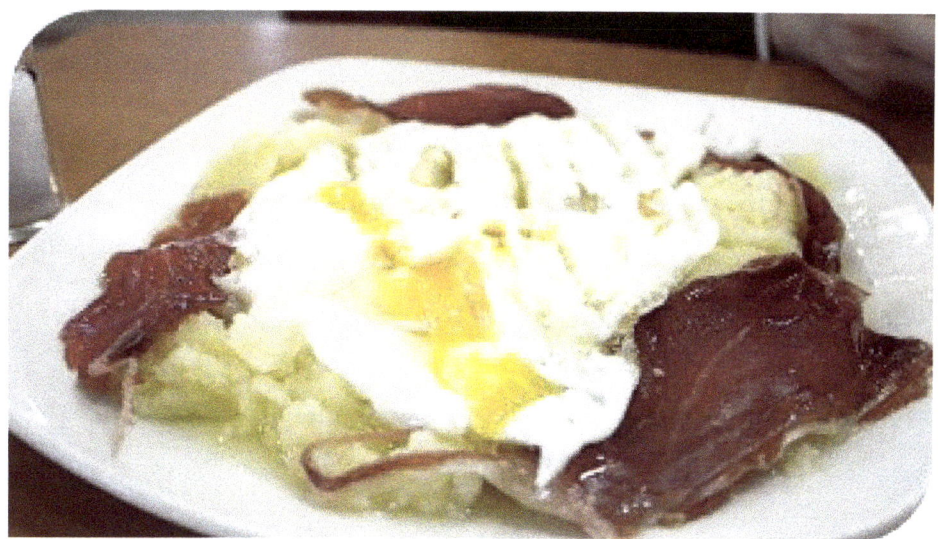

YUMMY

Ingredients

- 2-3 potatoes
- 1 onion
- 2 peppers
- ½ lb. chorizo or ham
- Salt
- Extra Virgin olive oil

Steps to Cook

1. Peel and wash the potatoes.

2. Cut them and put them in the bucket with a tablespoon of olive oil.

3. Once the potatoes are in, program the fryer for 25 minutes at 180ºC

4. When the time is up to 10 minutes, add the peppers that you have previously washed and cut.

5. In the last 3 minutes add the chorizo or ham.

6. After three minutes you have your potatoes ready.

7. Poach or grill eggs and break them on top of the potatoes.

Nutritional Information

- Calories: 1429
- Carbohydrates: 48g
- Fat: 131g
- Protein: 20g
- Sugar: 4g
- Cholesterol: 257mg

Air Fryer Cookbook

Omelette

• Servings: 4 • Preparation time: 30 minutes • Cook time: 20 minutes •

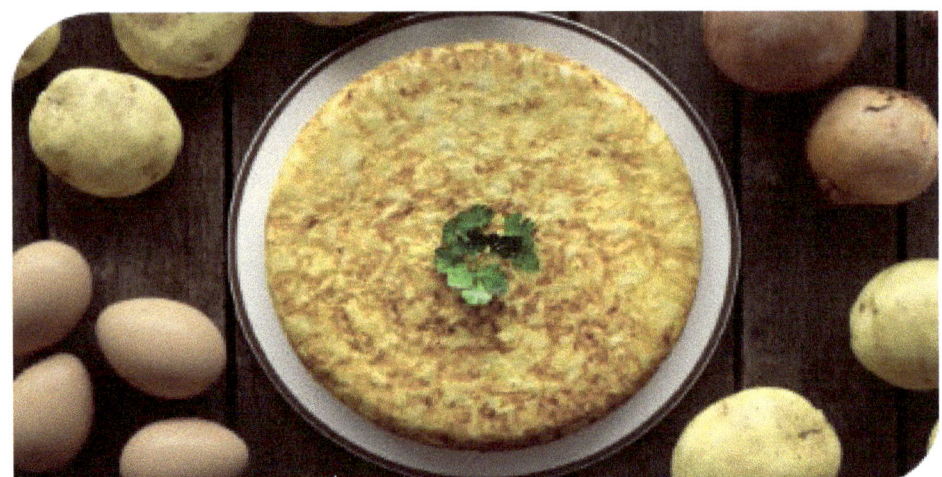

VERY EASY

Ingredients

- 6 potatoes
- 1 tbsp. oil
- Salt to taste
- 7 eggs

Steps to Cook

1. Peel and chop the potatoes.

2. Wash them well to remove the starch.

3. In a bowl, add a tablespoon of oil and mix well with the potatoes - this will prevent them from sticking and will keep them hydrated.

4. Put the potatoes in the fryer and cook at 180ºC for about 30 minutes.

5. Stir them every 5-10 min to make them even, if you don't have an automatic mixing system. If you have to remove them by hand, you may have to add a few more minutes to the time due to the loss of heat.

6. When you move them add the salt, so that it mixes well.

7. Beat the eggs.

8. When the potatoes are ready, remove them. Add the beaten egg.

9. Put the potato and egg mixture in the fryer. On Manuel, cook for 6-8 minutes at 130ºF.

....

Nutritional Information

- Calories: 323
- Carbohydrates: 1.4g
- Fat: 25g
- Protein: 21g
- Sugar: 0.6g
- Cholesterol: 625mg

Stuffed Potato

• Servings: 4• Preparation time: 30 minutes • Cook time: 20 minutes •

BUDGET FRIENDLY

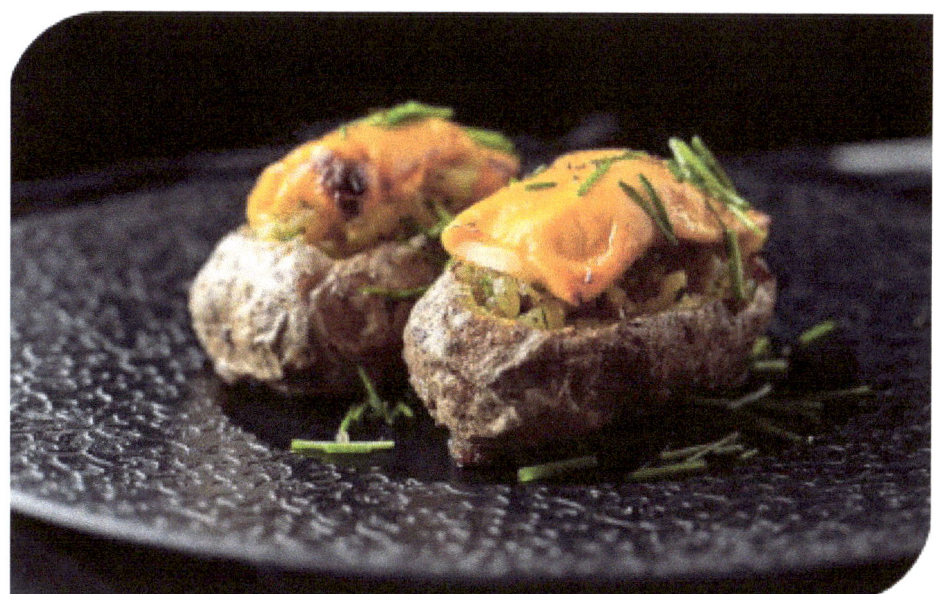

Ingredients

- 5.2 oz. Potatoes
- ½ cup Ham
- ½ cup Cheese
- Olive oil
- Salt
- Garlic powder

Steps to Cook

1. Cut your potato into strips but don't let the knife go all the way through.

2. Paint your potato with a little oil so it doesn't burn.

3. Add salt and pepper.

4. Put the potato to cook for 35 minutes at 180º without preheating the air fryer.

5. Fill each cut with ham and cheese to taste.

6. Put the potato back in for another 10 minutes at 180ºC.

Nutritional Information

- Calories: 130.6
- Carbohydrates: 22g
- Fat: 4g
- Protein: 3g
- Sugar: 3g
- Cholesterol: 75mg

Stuffed Portobello Mushrooms

• Servings: 4 • Preparation time: 5 minutes • Cook time: 15 minutes •

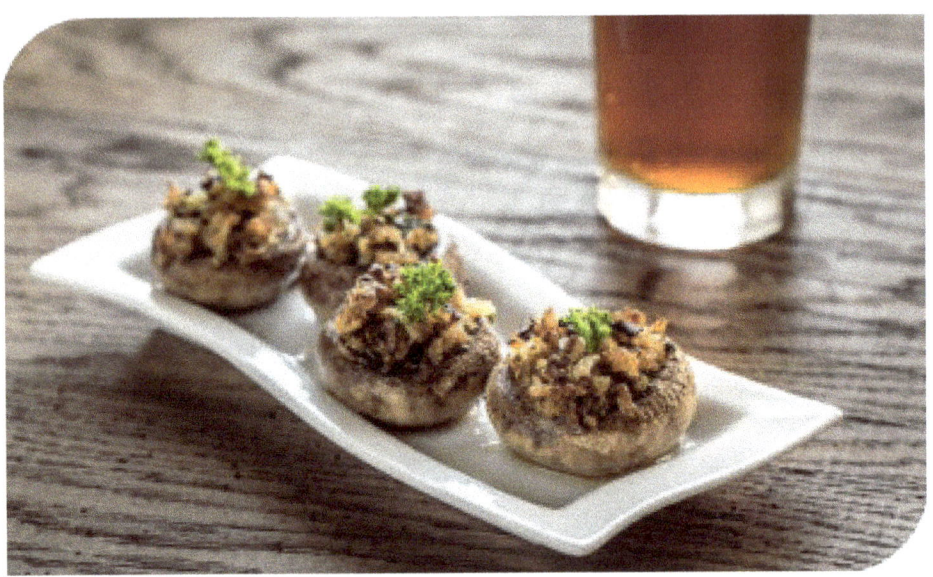

DELICIOUS

Ingredients

- 44-inch Portobello mushroom caps
- 4 tbsp. avocado oil
- 4 tbsp. balsamic vinegar
- Salt and pepper
- 1 cup grated mozzarella cheese
- 1 cup of greaves
- 1 cup grated Parmesan cheese
- ½ tbsp. of Italian seasoning
- 2 tbsp. melted butter

Steps to Cook

1. Preheat the air fryer to 170ºC. Brush the inside of each mushroom cap with avocado oil and balsamic vinegar. Season the inside of each with salt and pepper.

2. Sprinkle the mozzarella cheese in the center of the mushroom lids.

3. In a large bowl, combine the pork rinds, parmesan, Italian seasoning, and melted butter.

4. Spread the pork rind mixture evenly on the mushroom lids.

5. Spray the interior of the fryer with kitchen spray and place the mushrooms in the fryer 2 at a time (unless all 4 fit) and cook for 12 minutes or until the top is golden and crisp and the mushrooms are tender.

Nutritional Information

- Calories: 135.2
- Carbohydrates: 8.4g
- Fat: 5.5g
- Protein: 14.8g
- Sugar: 1.8g
- Cholesterol: 16.4mg

Antipasto Egg Rolls

• Servings: 4 • Preparation time: 5 minutes • Cook time: 12 minutes •

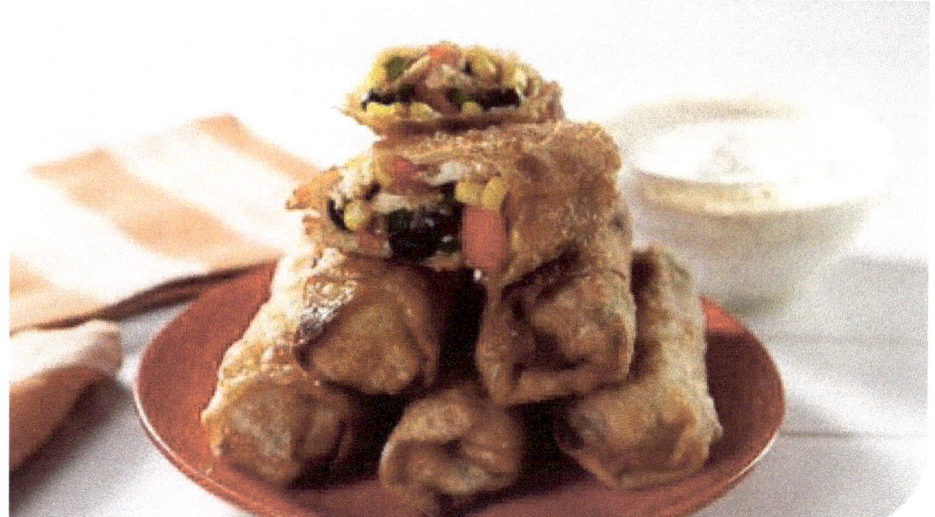

DELICIOUS

Ingredients

- 12 egg roll wrappers
- 12 slices of provolone
- 12 slices of deli ham
- 36 slices of pepperoni
- 1 cup crushed mozzarella
- 1 cup sliced pepperoncini
- Vegetable oil
- ¼ cup freshly grated parmesan
- 1 cup of Italian dressing, for serving

Steps to Cook

1. Lay an egg roll wrapper on a clean surface and place a slice of provolone in the center.

2. Top with a slice of ham, 3 slices of pepperoni, and a pinch of mozzarella and pepperoncini. Fold the bottom half and tightly fold the sides.

3. Roll it up gently, and then seal the fold with a couple of drops of water.

4. Cook in batches; cook the egg rolls at 390°F until golden brown, about 12 minutes, turning halfway.

Nutritional Information

- Calories: 148
- Carbohydrates: 19.4g
- Fat: 4.2g
- Protein: 9.1g
- Sugar: 4g
- Cholesterol: 120mg

Avocado With Bacon

• Servings: 4 • Preparation time: 5 minutes • Cook time: 15 minutes •

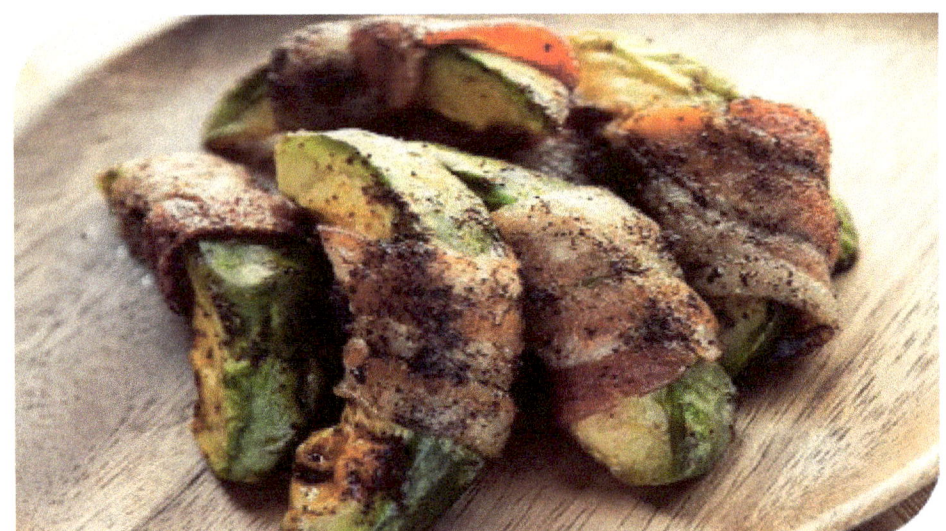

HIGH CALORIES

Ingredients

- 3 avocados
- 24 slices of bacon
- Quarter spoon of ranch dressing sauce

Steps to Cook

1. Cut each avocado into 8 wedges of the same size.
2. Wrap each wedge with a strip of bacon, cutting the bacon if necessary.
3. Fill the fryer basket in a single layer.
4. Cook 400 degrees for 8 minutes until the bacon is cooked and crispy.
5. Serve it hot with the sauce

....

Nutritional Information

- Calories: 810
- Carbohydrates: 53g
- Fat: 51g
- Protein: 36g
- Sugar: 7g
- Cholesterol: 85mg

Breakfast Pizza

• Servings:1-2• Preparation time: 5 minutes• Cook time: 8 minutes •

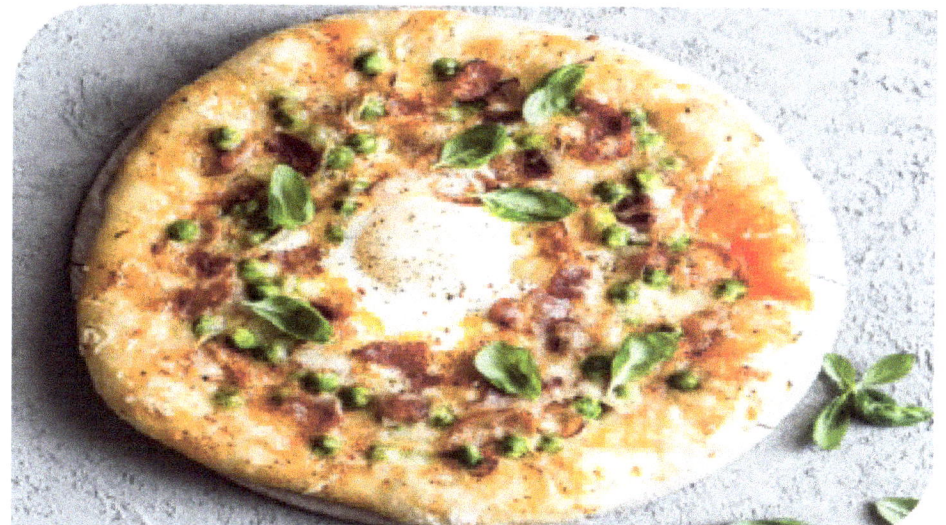

DELICIOUS

Ingredients

- 2 tsp olive oil
- 1 pizza dough (178 mm)
- 1 oz. semi-dry mozzarella
- 2 slices of smoked ham
- 1 egg
- ½ tsp chopped coriander

Steps to Cook

1. Brush the olive oil over the pizza dough.

2. Add the mozzarella and smoked ham to the dough.

3. Select Preheat on the Air Fryer, set to 350°F.

4. Place the pizza in the preheated air fryer and bake for 8 minutes at 350°F. Remove the baskets after 5 minutes and break the egg onto the pizza.

5. Return the baskets to the fryer and finish cooking. Garnish with chopped coriander and serve.

Nutritional Information

- Calories: 354
- Carbohydrates: 23g
- Fat: 21g
- Protein: 17g
- Sugar:1.8g
- Cholesterol: 184m

BBQ Bacon

• Servings: 2 • Preparation time: 2 minutes • Cook time: 8 minutes •

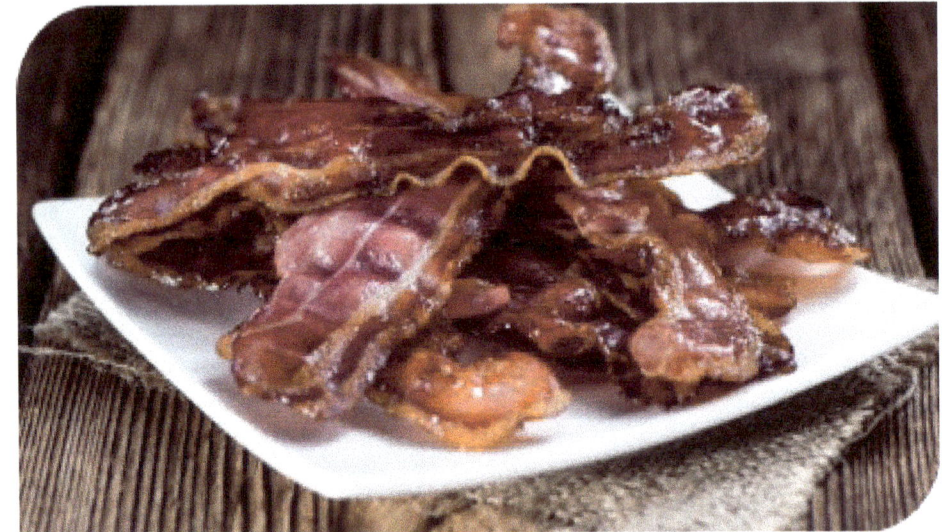

SWEET AND SPICY

Ingredients

- 1/3 oz. brown sugar
- 1 tsp chili powder
- 1 tsp cumin powder
- ¼ tsp cayenne pepper
- 4 slices bacon, halved

Steps to Cook

1. Mix the seasonings.

2. Sprinkle the seasoning over the bacon until completely covered. Reserve.

3. Select Preheat on the Air Fryer, set to 320°F and press Start/Pause.

4. Place the bacon in the preheated air fryer.

5. Select Bacon and press Start/Pause.

Nutritional Information

- Calories: 195
- Carbohydrates: 23g
- Fat: 7g
- Protein: 10g
- Sugar: 0g
- Cholesterol: 40mg

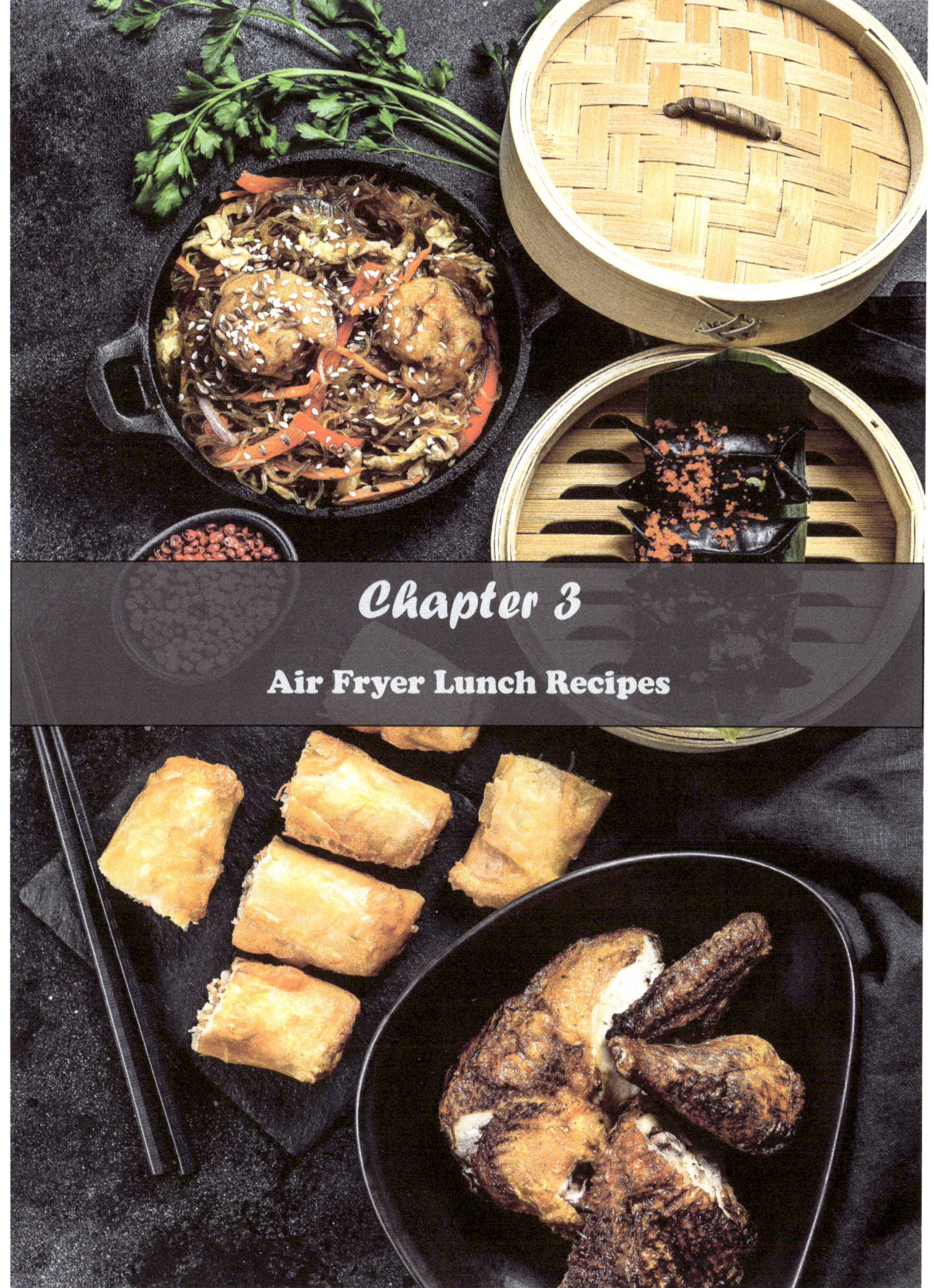

Chapter 3

Air Fryer Lunch Recipes

Chicken Thighs

• Servings: 1-2 • Preparation time: 5 minutes • Cook time: 8 minutes •

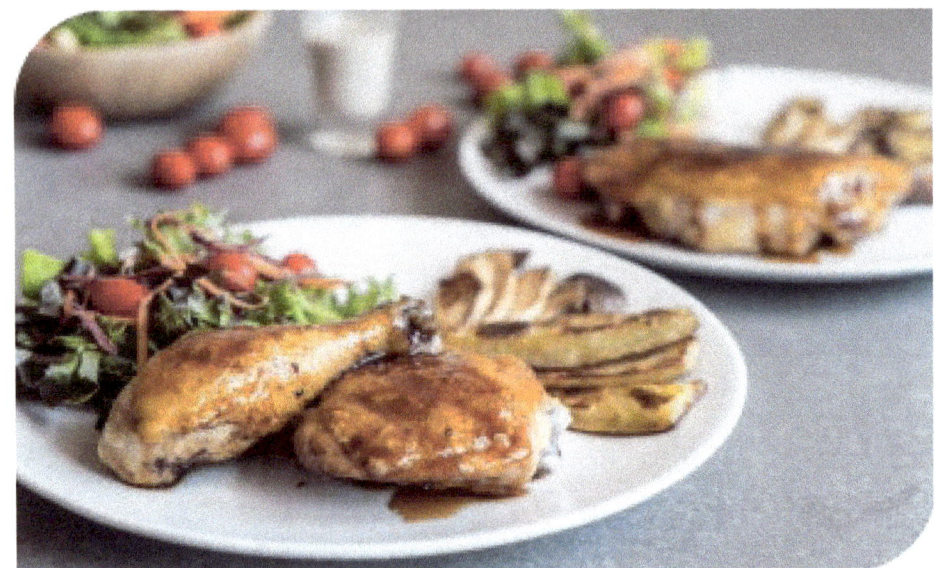

TOOTHSOME

Ingredients

- 4 chicken thighs, trimmed from excess fat and skin
- ½ tsp salt
- 1 tsp of paprika
- 1 tsp of garlic powder
- ½ tsp of oregano
- ½ tsp onion powder

Steps to Cook

1. Preheat your fryer to 190ºC for 5 minutes. After preheating, spray with cooking spray.

2. Add chicken thighs to a large zippered bag or bowl with a lid. Top with salt, paprika, garlic powder, oregano, and onion powder. Shake to cover.

3. Place the chicken thighs in the fryer, skin-side down, for 12 minutes.

4. Turn the chicken thighs upside-down and cook for an additional 10 minutes. If you want your chicken drumsticks to be super crispy. Cook in 4 minute increments to get your desired crisp.

5. The thighs are made when an internal meat thermometer reads 70ºC. To serve.

Nutritional Information

- Calories: 135
- Carbohydrates: 0g
- Fat: 8.45g
- Protein: 13.67g
- Sugar: 0g
- Cholesterol: 51mg

Garlic Shrimp

• Servings: 2 • Preparation time: 5 minutes • Cook time: 10 minutes •

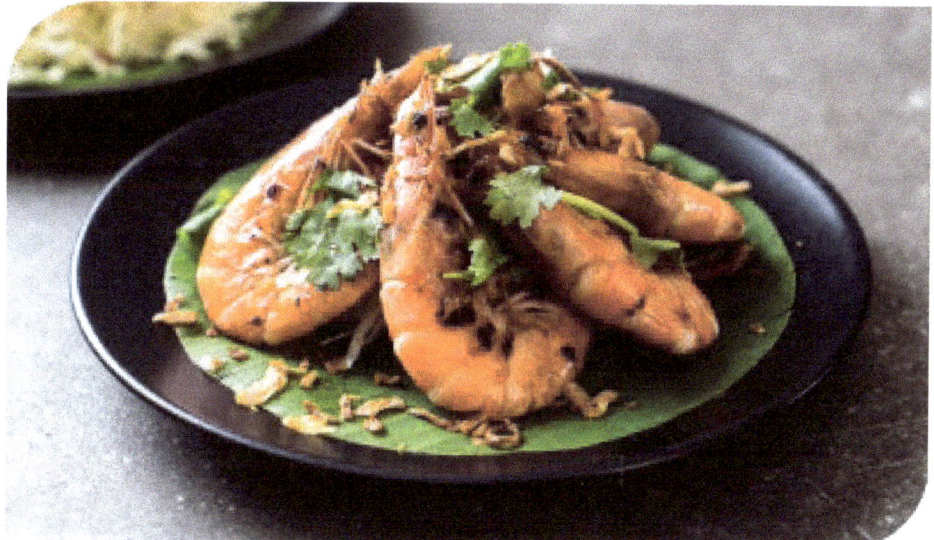

CRUNCHY

Ingredients

- 1 pound shrimp, peeled and deveined
- 1 tsp of garlic powder
- 1 tbsp of oil
- ½ tsp salt
- ½ tsp of pepper

Steps to Cook

1. In a medium bowl, place the shrimp, garlic powder, avocado oil, salt, and pepper. Mix to combine.

2. Place the shrimp in your deep fryer. Adjust at 100ºC for 10 minutes. No need to shake in half. The 10 minutes is the perfect time for the giant shrimp, but if the shrimp are smaller, you would need to cook for a shorter period of time.

3. Serve.

....

Nutritional Information

- Calories: 224
- Carbohydrates: 1.3g
- Fat: 10g
- Protein: 32g
- Sugar: 0.1g
- Cholesterol: 263mg

Air Fryer Cookbook

Salmon

• Servings: 2-4 • Preparation time: 5 minutes • Cook time: 10 minutes •

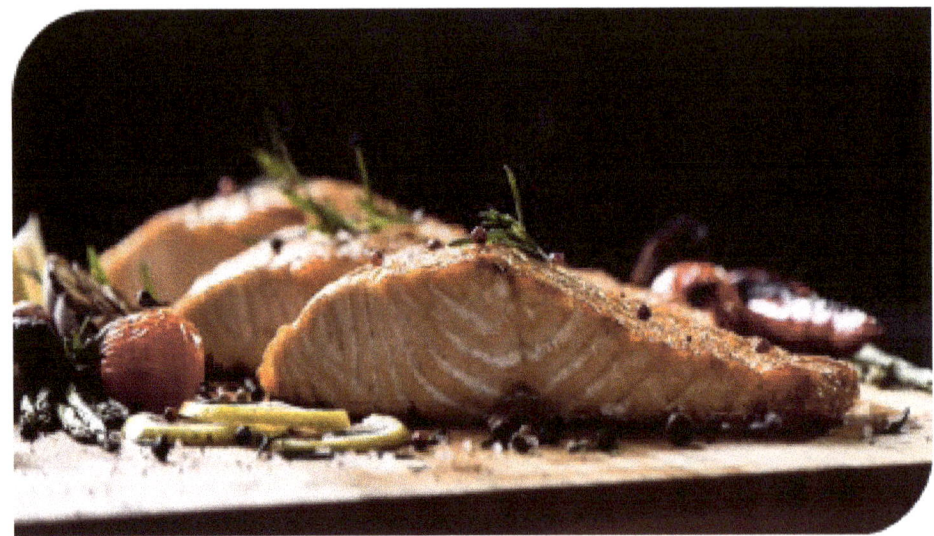

EASY & QUICK

Ingredients

- 2 boneless salmon fillets
- 2 tbsp of oil
- 2 tbsp of lime juice
- ½ tsp chili powder
- ½ tsp ground cumin
- ½ tsp garlic powder
- Salt and pepper to taste

Steps to Cook

1. Mix the oil, lime juice, chili powder, ground cumin, garlic powder, salt, and pepper in a small bowl.

2. Mix well to make sure all of your ingredients come together to make a paste.

3. Use a brush to spread the mixture all over the sides of the salmon fillet.

4. Place in the fryer.

5. Cook at 200ºC for 10 minutes. Or cook until desired temperature is reached.

Nutritional Information

- Calories: 179
- Carbohydrates: 0g
- Fat: 10.43g
- Protein: 19.93g
- Sugar: 0g
- Cholesterol: 46mg

Pork Loin

• Servings: 1 • Preparation time: 2 minutes • Cook time: 10 minutes •

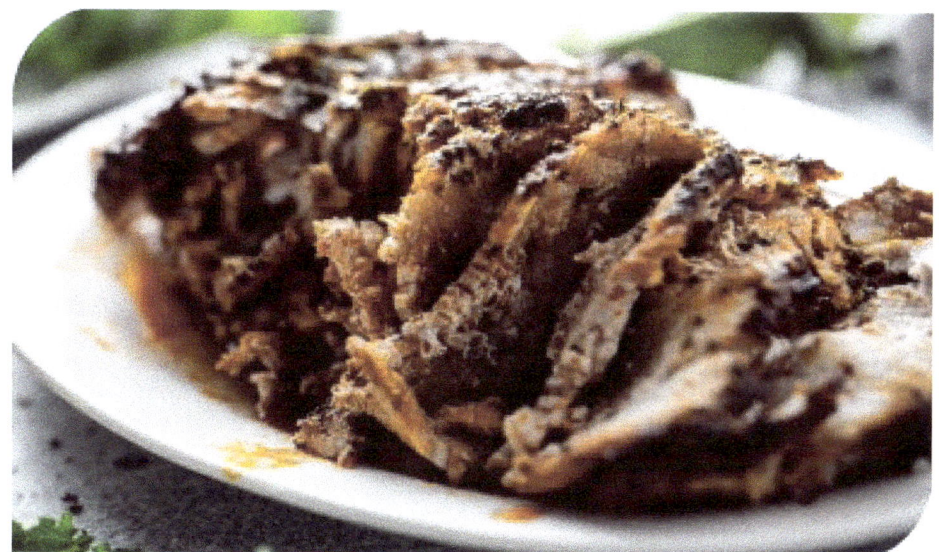

Ingredients

- 1 pound whole pork loin
- 1 tsp of garlic powder
- 1 tsp of cumin
- 1 tsp of oregano
- 1 tsp dried thyme
- 2 garlic cloves, minced
- 1 tbsp of oil
- 1 tsp salt
- ½ tsp of pepper

Steps to Cook

1. In a small bowl, combine all the spices, salt, pepper and oil to create dough.

2. Place the pork loin on a cutting board and cover everything with the dough.

3. Place in the fryer and cook at 90°C for 20 minutes or until the internal temperature reaches 60°C with a meat thermometer.

Nutritional Information

- Calories: 55.3
- Carbohydrates: 0g
- Fat: 2.2g
- Protein: 8.4g
- Sugar: 0g
- Cholesterol: 22.1mg

Air Fryer Cookbook

Garlic hake

• Servings: 4 • Preparation time: 5 minutes • Cook time: 10 minutes •

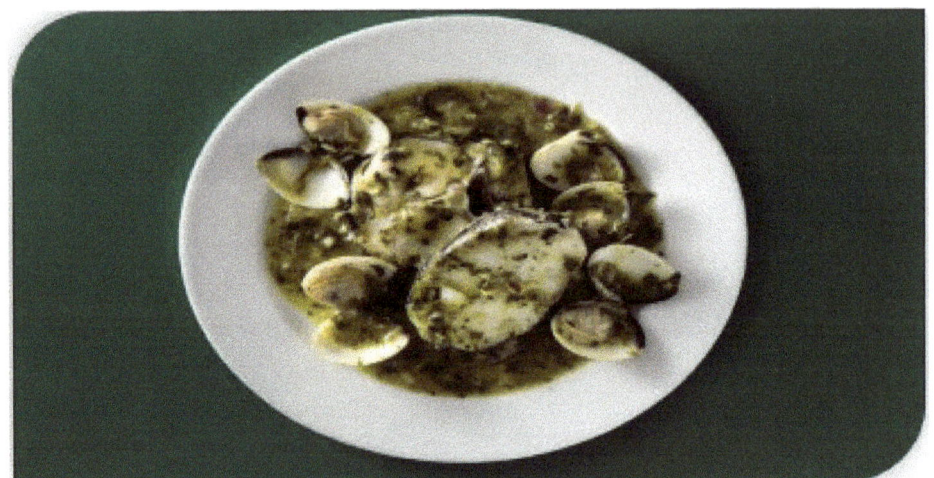

RICH

Ingredients

- 1 or 2 fillets per person
- 2 garlic cloves
- Parsley
- Extra virgin olive oil
- Salt

Steps to Cook

1. If the hake fillets are frozen, they should be allowed to thaw.

2. Once thawed, they are dried well with kitchen paper.

3. We place the fish in the upper tray of our fryer or in the bowl but without the central shovel.

4. Add salt, garlic and a drizzle of extra virgin olive oil.

5. We select the fish program in Actifry 2 in 1 or also 10 minutes in normal.

6. When the program ends our fish will be ready..

Nutritional Information

- Calories: 114
- Carbohydrates: 1.3g
- Fat: 1.3g
- Protein: 25.4g
- Sugar: 0g
- Cholesterol: 51mg

Sausages

• Servings: 2 • Preparation time: 2 minutes • Cook time: 10 minutes •

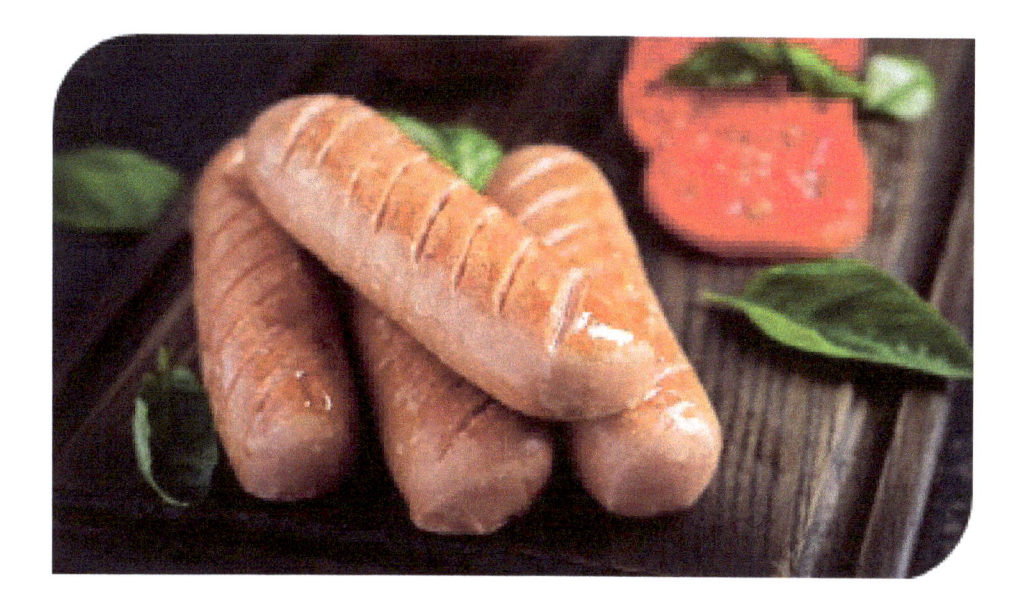

Ingredients

- 4 fresh or frozen sausages
- Olive oil

Steps to Cook

1. If the sausages are frozen they are removed and placed directly in the fryer.

2. To defrost them and remove part of the fat, they are boiled for 5-10 minutes.

3. When they are punctured to remove the remaining fat. In a bowl put the sausages and add a spoon of oil and mix well.

4. Add the sausages in the fryer.

5. Program at 190ºC for about 10 minutes.

6. After ten minutes you already have the sausages ready to accompany any dish of vegetables, rice, potatoes, etc.

Nutritional Information

- Calories: 186
- Carbohydrates: 2g
- Fat: 14g
- Protein: 7g
- Sugar: 1g
- Cholesterol: 46mg

Air Fryer Cookbook

Fried Fish

• Servings: 1 • Preparation time: 5 minutes • Cook time: 5 minutes •

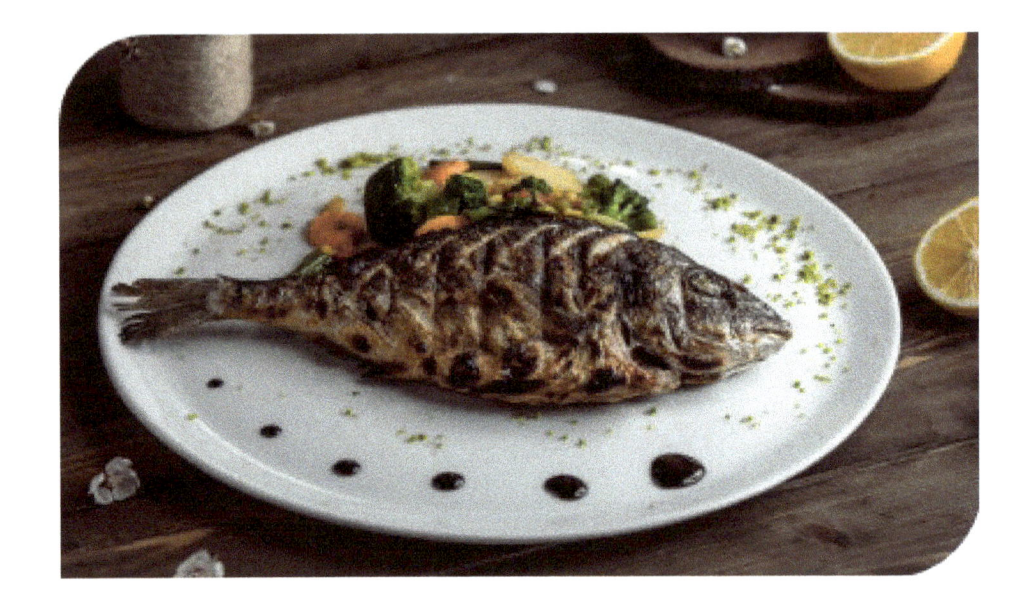

CRUNCHY

Ingredients

- 1 Raw fish, hake sticks or frozen fish figurines
- Oil
- Salt

Steps to Cook

1. We clean and wash the fresh fish.

2. Dry with kitchen paper, salt a little and flour.

3. Place the fish in the fryer, add a spoon of oil and select the time at 150ºC.

4. In the case of hake leave it 15 minutes on each side.

If you are going to prepare anchovies, they need 5 minutes on each side.

Nutritional Information

- Calories: 199
- Carbohydrates: 7g
- Fat: 12g
- Protein: 16g
- Sugar: 0.6g
- Cholesterol: 62mg

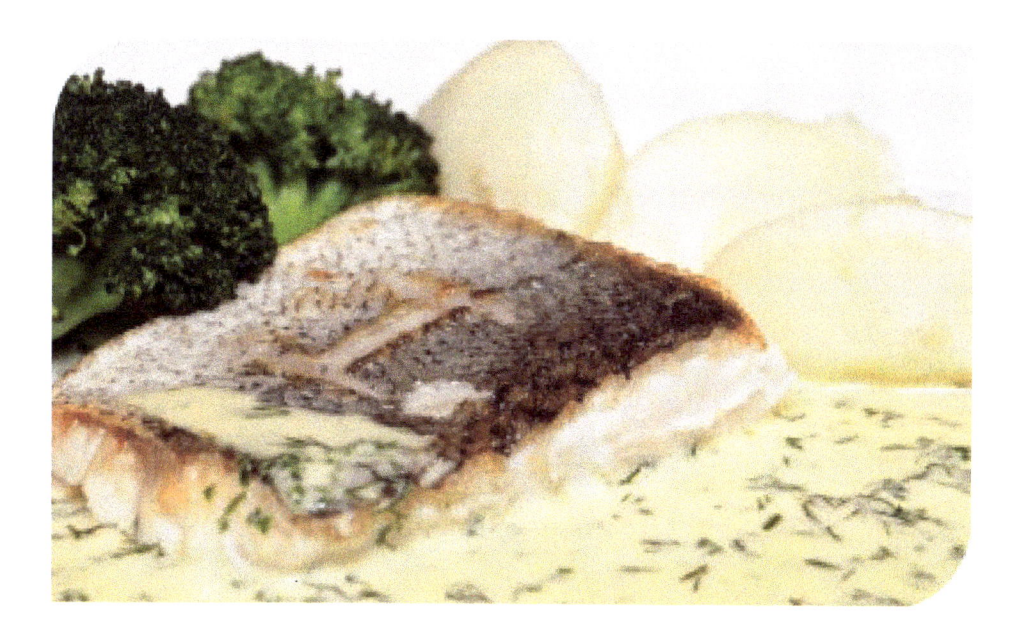

FANTASTIC

Hake With Lemon

• Servings: 1 • Preparation time:30 minutes • Cook time: 20 minutes •

Ingredients

- 1 fillet of hake
- 4 cloves of garlic
- 1 large lemon
- Salt
- olive oil
- 1 kg of potatoes
- Parsley

Steps to Cook

1. Peel and wash the potatoes. Cut them to the cane as equal as possible.

2. Put the potatoes in the fryer and add a tablespoon of oil. Program the fryer for 30 minutes by giving the +, then give the 2 × 1 until the fish symbol appears and press start. Once the time is selected, the fryer starts, what will work is the bottom part where the potatoes are. When it is 10 minutes to finish, it will warn you and you will have to open and place the tray on top where you have previously placed fish.

3. The hake fillets, before putting them add the lemon juice, a tablespoon of oil, salt and a little parsley.

4. Once everything is set, start it. When the time is up, it warns you again and take out the hake and the potatoes.

....

Nutritional Information

- Calories: 159
- Carbohydrates: 14g
- Fat: 8.1g
- Protein: 9.5g
- Sugar: 1g
- Cholesterol: 46mg

Air Fryer Cookbook

Meatballs

• Servings: 4 • Preparation time: 5 minutes • Cook time: 23minutes •

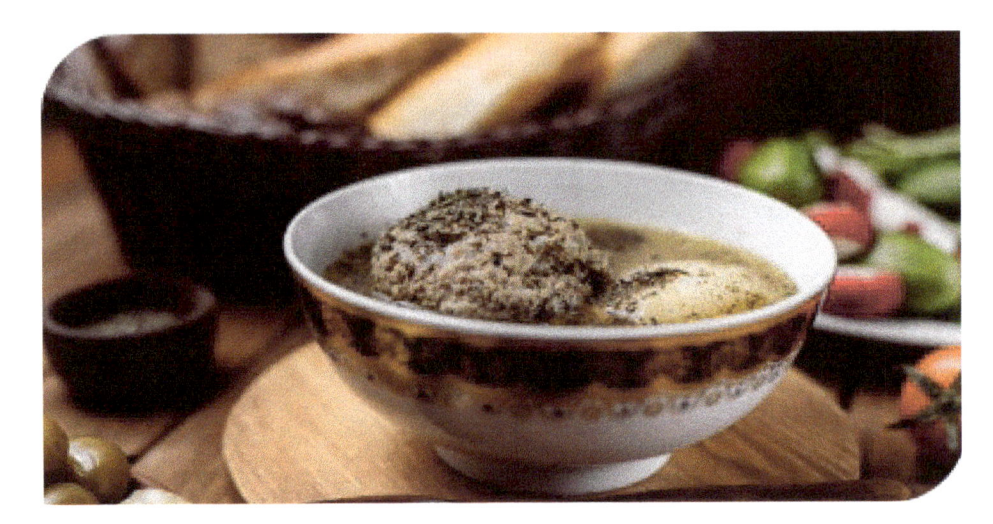

EXTRAORDINARY

Ingredients

For meatballs:
- 1 lb of minced meat
- 2 eggs
- Garlic
- Parsley
- Bread crumbs
- A bit of milk
- Salt

For the sauce:
- Onion
- A glass of water
- A glass of broth
- olive oil
- A tablespoon of flour
- Salt

Steps to Cook

1. The first step is to prepare the meat. Put the meat, the parsley, the egg, the salt and the garlic in a bowl, mix everything well.

2. Add the breadcrumbs and milk and mix everything again. Once the meatball meat ready, shape it.

3. Put them in the fryer without oil and put the corresponding time, depending on the model of your fryer at 150°C for 25 minutes. To avoid burning from time to time you can give them a few laps.

4. While the meatballs are being made prepare the sauce, for that in a frying pan fry the onion washed and cut into small pieces.

5. When the onion is poached add the rest of the ingredients to the sauce.

6. Start with the flour that also going to fry a little.

7. Add the broth, water and salt and let it reduce until you have the desired texture for our sauce.

8. When you have the sauce add the meatballs to the sauce, we let all the flavors mix well and ready.

Nutritional Information

- Calories: 57
- Carbohydrates: 2.12g
- Fat: 3.69g
- Protein: 3.47g
- Sugar: 0.42g
- Cholesterol: 21mg

Chicken Wings With Barbecue Sauce

• Servings: 4 • Preparation time: 30 minutes • Cook time: 20 minutes •

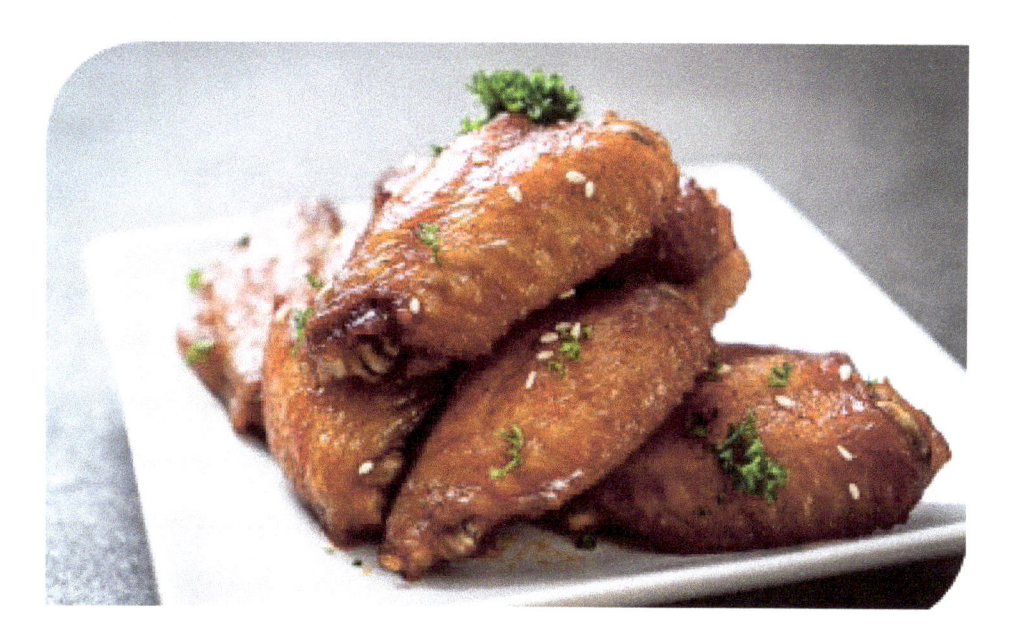

TASTEFUL

Ingredients

- 12 chicken wings
- Salt
- Ground pepper
- 2 tablespoons of olive oil
- 6 tablespoons of barbecue sauce

Steps to Cook

1. In a bowl we put the olive oil together with the barbecue sauce and mix well until everything is well linked.

2. Next we salt the wings and place them in the bowl of the deep fryer without oil.

3. With the help of a silicone brush paint the wings with the mixture of the barbecue sauce and the oil.

4. Once the wings are ready we select 20 minutes at 180ºC. After this time check that the wings are well made, if they are ready serve them. If you see that they are not, put them to cook a little more.

Nutritional Information

- Calories: 180
- Carbohydrates: 1g
- Fat: 12g
- Protein: 18g
- Sugar: 0g
- Cholesterol: 95mg

Air Fryer Cookbook

Rice With Squid

• Servings: 4 • Preparation time: 45 minutes • Cook time: 50 minutes •

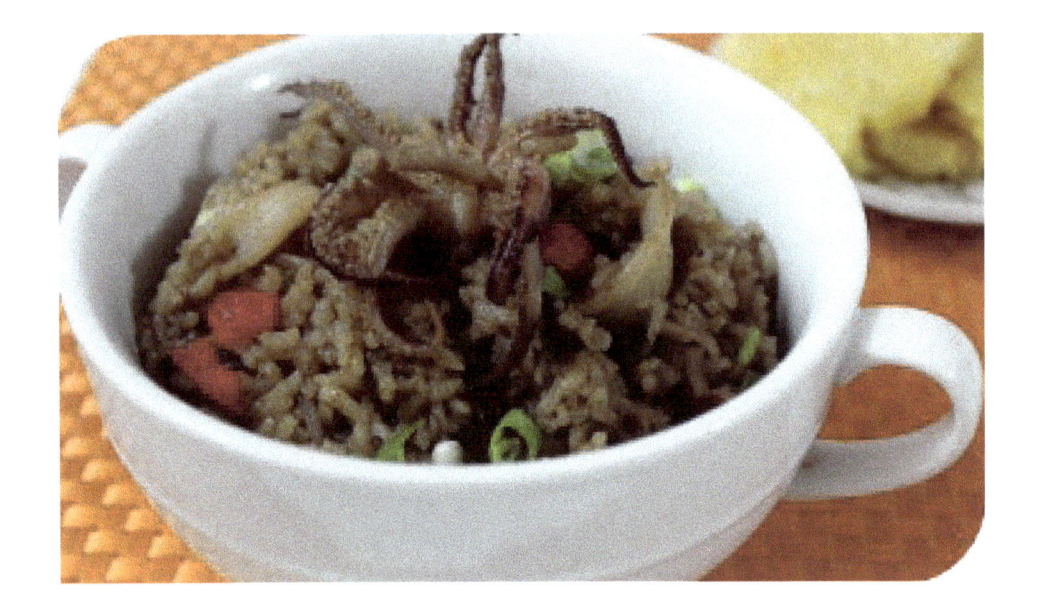

DELICIOUS

Ingredients

- 1 onion
- 2 garlic cloves
- Half a spoon of paprika
- 3 ½ cup chicken broth
- 7 oz. of rice
- 1 tbsp fried tomato
- 1 tbsp of oil
- 7 oz. of prawns
- 7 oz. of squid
- Salt

Steps to Cook

1. Put the oil, the clean and chopped onion and the chopped garlic in the fryer. Program 4 minutes more or less at 150°C.

2. Once the onion and garlic are browned, add the rice, the paprika, the tomato, the chicken stock, salt and mix everything. Program the fryer for 35 minutes.

3. Once the time has passed, add the chopped shrimp and squid and add another 10 minutes.

Nutritional Information

- Calories: 194.9
- Carbohydrates: 38.7g
- Fat: 10.1g
- Protein: 11.1g
- Sugar: 0g
- Cholesterol: 0mg

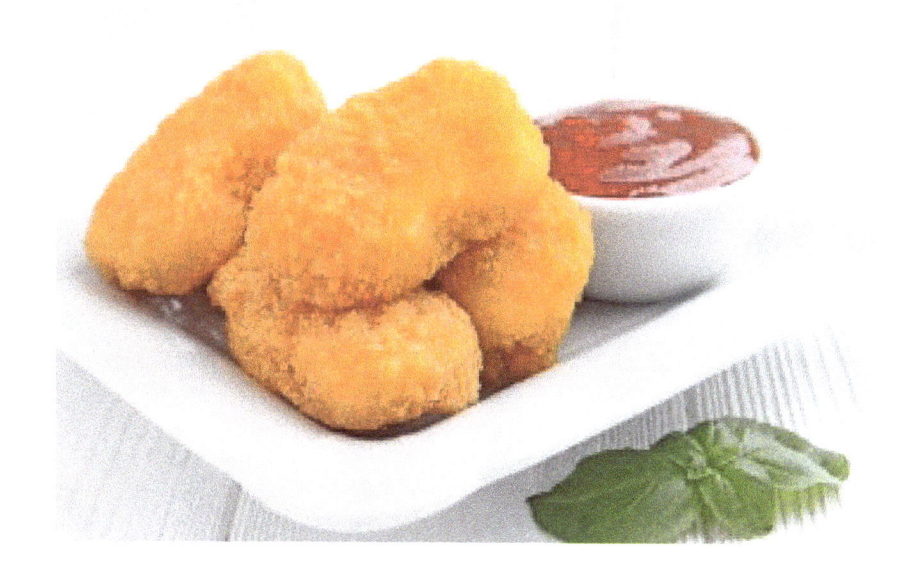

ZESTY

Nuggets

• Servings: 6 • Preparation time: 45 minutes • Cook time: 25 minutes •

Ingredients

- 1 pound of chicken breast in small pieces
- 2 garlic cloves
- fresh parsley
- Salt
- 50 gr bread crumbs or sliced bread
- 1 ½ oz. of milk
- 4 cheeses

To coat:
- I beaten egg
- garlic and parsley breadcrumbs

Steps to Cook

1. Chop the breast with the help of a food processor or mincer. Mix the garlic, parsley and salt in the mortar and add the meat.

2. In a bowl soak the bread with the milk, once wet, crush it with the help of a fork, and add the cheese and meat.

3. Mix everything well until all the ingredients are well incorporated. Once the dough is ready it is time to shape the nuggets. For that, form balls and then crush them. If while you shape the nuggets you see that they stick to your hands, you can smear your hands with a little oil.

4. Once the nuggets are done, pass them through egg and breadcrumbs and they are ready to fry and serve.

Nutritional Information

- Calories: 49
- Carbohydrates: 2.4g
- Fat: 3.3g
- Protein: 2.5g
- Sugar: 0g
- Cholesterol: 8.8mg

Keto Style KFC Chicken

• Servings: 4 • Preparation time: 5 minutes • Cook time: 40 minutes •

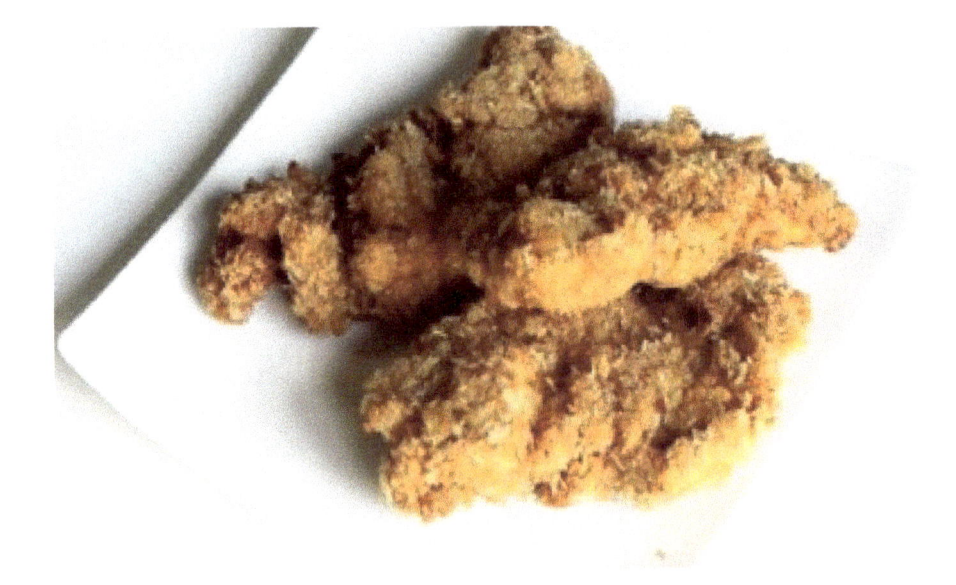

Ingredients

- 4 Chicken pieces
- ½ cup almond flour
- 1 tablespoon psyllium husk
- to taste cayenne pepper
- to taste thyme
- to taste oregano
- to taste cumin
- to taste garlic powder
- to taste Salt

Steps to Cook

1. Mix the flour and the spaces in a ziploc bag.
2. Each piece of chicken is placed separately and the bag is shaken.
3. Do it with each piece and put it in the fryer at 400ºF for 20 minutes on each side.

Nutritional Information

- Calories: 80
- Carbohydrates: 0g
- Fat: 4g
- Protein: 11g
- Sugar: 0g
- Cholesterol: 157mg

Beef Pancakes With Spinach

• Servings: 5-7 • Preparation time: 2 h 5 minutes • Cook time: 25 minutes •

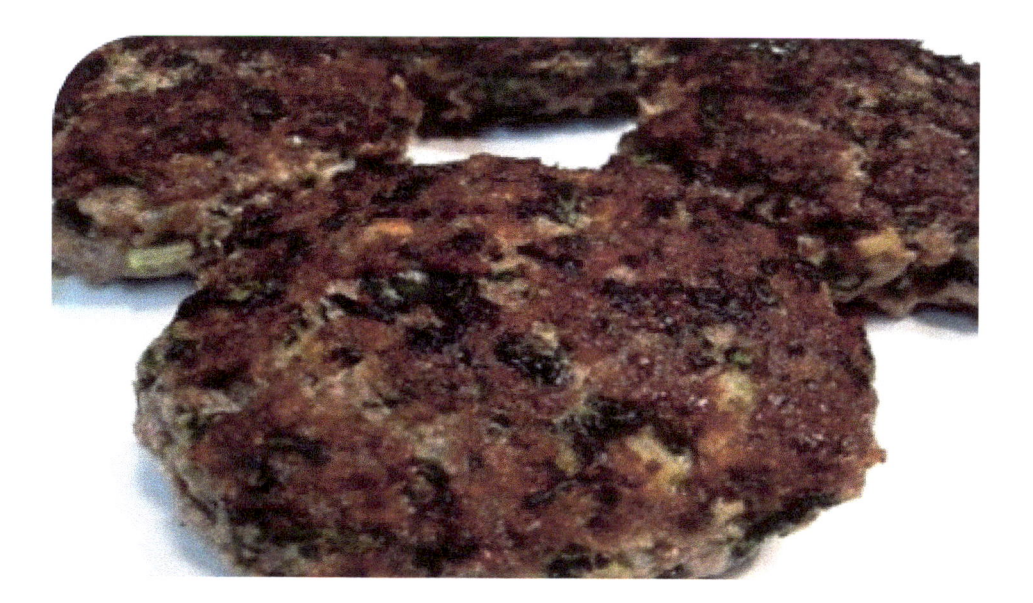

CRISPY

Ingredients

- 1 pound ground beef
- Tomato to taste
- Onion to taste
- Green chili to taste
- Spinach to taste
- Mustard to taste
- Worcestershire sauce
- Beef consommé to taste
- 1 egg

Steps to Cook

1. Chop the tomato, spinach, onion, green chili. Mix it with Worcestershire sauce, broth and mustard.

2. Add the meat and mix until fully integrated. Leave it like this for 2 hours. Before putting it into the fryer, add the egg and the breadcrumb and mix it.

3. Prepare your pancakes and put them in the fryer for 15 minutes at 360°F without any additional fat.

4. After 10 minutes open the fryer and turn the pancakes so that they cook evenly on both sides. Ready.

Nutritional Information

- Calories: 130.9
- Carbohydrates: 3.6g
- Fat: 8.8g
- Protein: 9.8g
- Sugar: 0.3g
- Cholesterol: 31.1mg

Air Fryer Cookbook

Sweet and sour pork cutlet

• Servings: 5 • Preparation time: 3h 5 minutes • Cook time: 29 minutes •

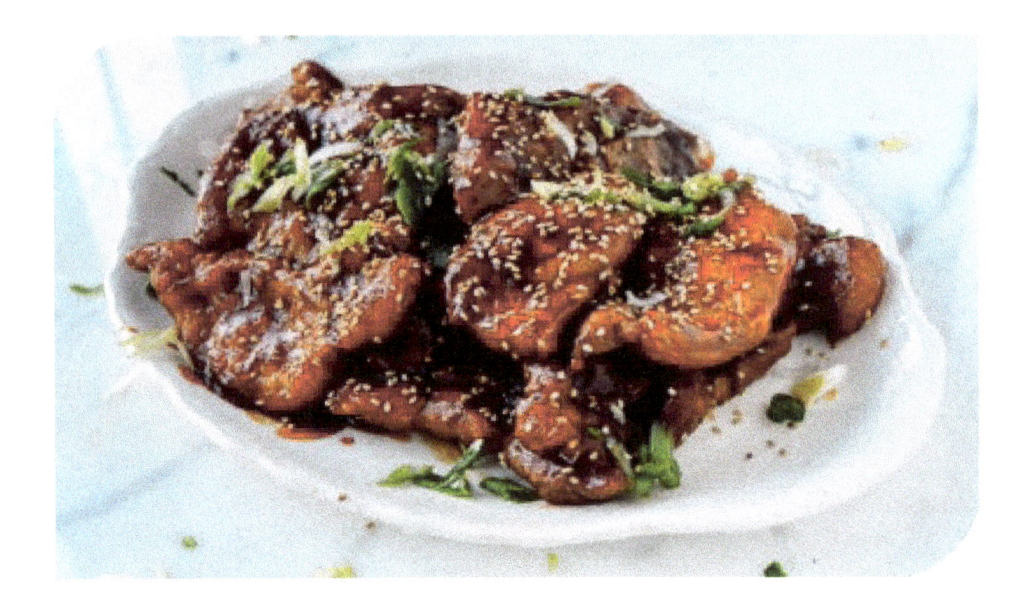

SWEET

Ingredients

- 1 pound regular pork chops
- Honey to taste
- Chicken broth (no rib) to taste
- Ketchup to taste
- White vinegar to taste

Steps to Cook

1. Mix all the ingredients in a sufficient quantity to marinate all the meat. Prepare the meat at least 3 hours before so that it absorbs the flavor.

2. Place it in the air fryer at 400ºF for 14 minutes then flip it for an additional 5 minutes. No additional fat is added.

3. Once it is golden brown ready to serve.

4. You can add applesauce if you like.

Nutritional Information

- Calories: 504.9
- Carbohydrates: 35.3g
- Fat: 25.7g
- Protein: 31.3g
- Sugar: 8.7g
- Cholesterol: 71.2mg

Pumpkins With Parmesan Cheese

• Servings: 4 • Preparation time: 35 minutes • Cook time: 10 minutes •

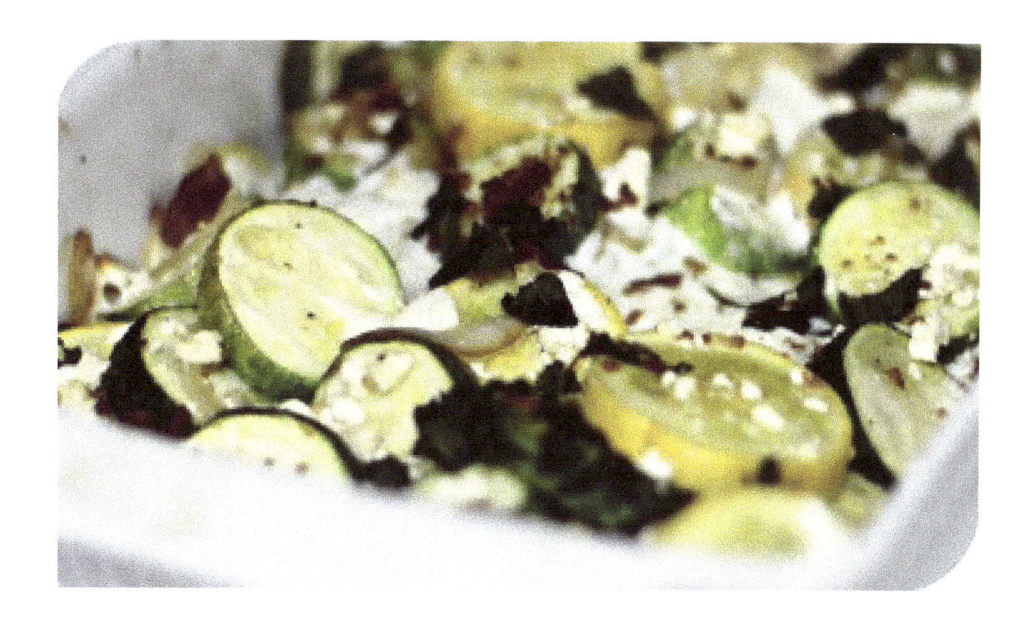

FANTASTIC

Ingredients

- 2 pumpkins
- 1 cup parmesan cheese, ground
- ½ cup almond flour
- Garlic powder to taste
- Paprika to taste
- Pepper to taste
- Italian spices to taste
- 2 eggs
- Salt to taste

Steps to Cook

1. Cut the pumpkins and salt them, reserve for 10 minutes, then rinse them.

2. Beat the egg in a bowl.

3. Mix the Parmesan cheese and flour with the spices.

4. Pass the vegetables through the egg, then through the cheese and arrange in a pan in the fryer, bake at 300ºF for 15 minutes.

Nutritional Information

- Calories: 68.2
- Carbohydrates: 4.6g
- Fat: 7.7g
- Protein: 4.9g
- Sugar: 0.8g
- Cholesterol: 58.4mg

Air Fryer Cookbook

Chicken With Mustard

• Servings: 1 • Preparation time: 5 minutes • Cook time: 40 minutes •

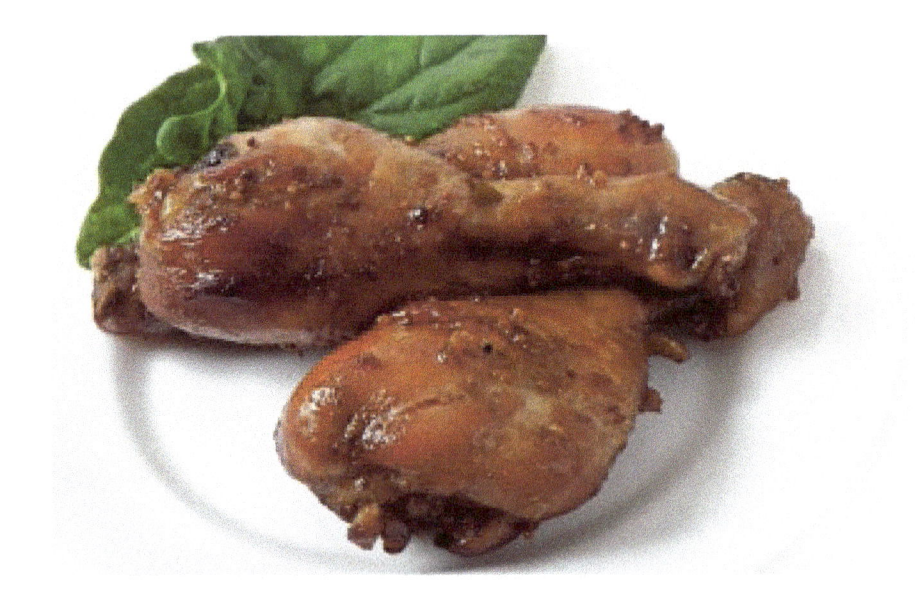

DELICIOUS

Ingredients

- 3 pieces chicken

Cover:

- ¼ cup Dijon mustard
- 1 tbsp minced garlic
- 4 tbsp apple cider vinegar
- ½ bunch coriander
- 1 tbsp erythritol
- 3 tbsp sunflower seeds
- Chambray onion for garnish

Steps to Cook

1. All the ingredients of the cover are mixed.

2. Each piece of chicken is passed through the cover, trying to make it completely covered; they are arranged in a mold for the fryer.

3. Put the chicken in the air fryer at 350ºF for 20 minutes on each side.

Nutritional Information

- Calories: 271.5
- Carbohydrates: 32g
- Fat: 6.9g
- Protein: 18.2g
- Sugar: 0.1g
- Cholesterol: 53.2mg

Lemon Pepper Chicken

• Servings: 2 • Preparation time: 5 minutes • Cook time: 40 minutes •

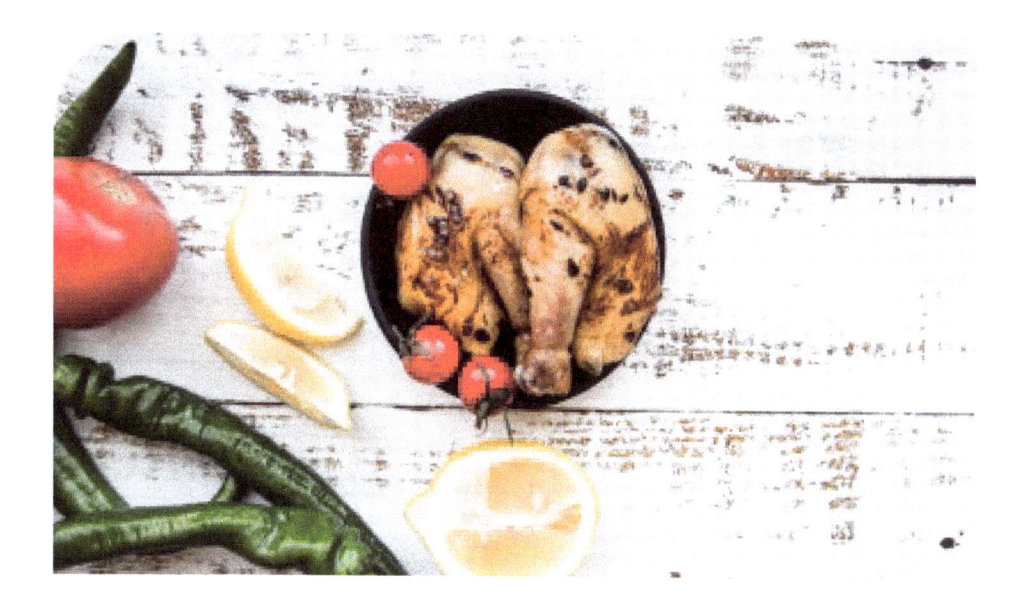

WONDERFUL

Ingredients

- 1 lb Chicken in pieces (with or without bone, as you wish)
- pepper-lemon to taste for seasoning

Steps to Cook

1. In a large bowl, generously mix chicken with lemon pepper to coat.

2. Put the chicken in the fryer and cook at 400ºF, 20 minutes on one side, flip the pieces over and another 20 minutes.

Nutritional Information

- Calories: 149.4
- Carbohydrates: 35g
- Fat: 1.7g
- Protein: 29.6g
- Sugar: 1.3g
- Cholesterol: 68.4mg

Air Fryer Cookbook

Roasted Fish

• Servings: 1-2 • Preparation time: 5 minutes • Cook time: 5 minutes •

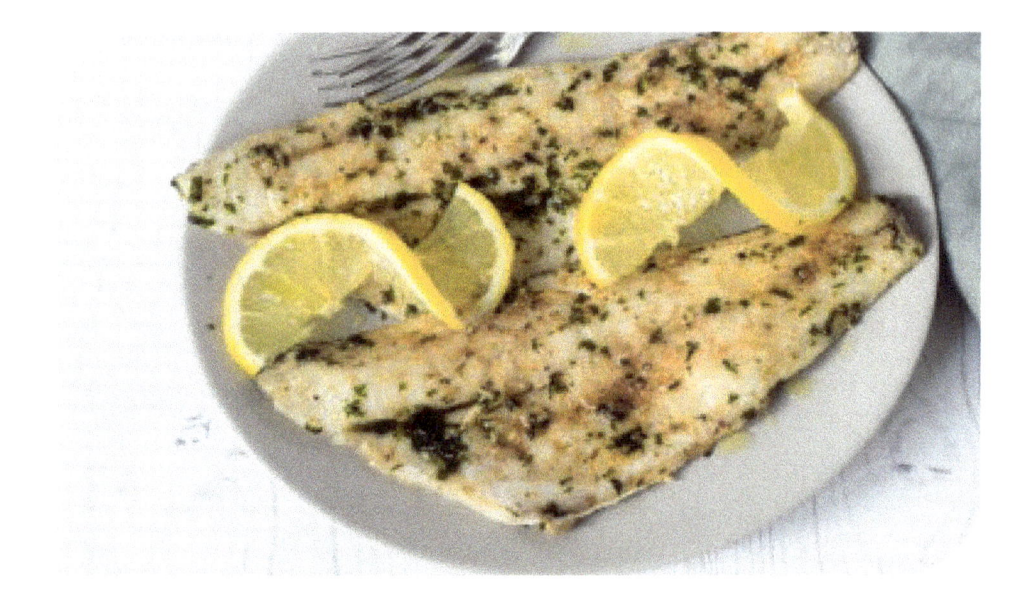

LOVELY

Ingredients

- Juice of 1 lemon
- 3 fish fillets
- 1 tbsp seasoning complete with achiote
- 1 tbsp minced garlic
- 1 tbsp ground onion
- Chickpea flour needed
- Water

Steps to Cook

1. Rinse the fish. And cut them into pieces. Dry with paper towels. Spread with the lemon and season.

2. In a bowl add the chickpea flour and little water to form a thick cream.

3 Coat the pieces of fish. Grease the pan of the fryer with oil and place the fish in the air fryer. Cook at 150ºC for 5 minutes.

Nutritional Information

- Calories: 165.1
- Carbohydrates: 19.4g
- Fat: 0.5g
- Protein: 25.9g
- Sugar: 0g
- Cholesterol: 50.6mg

Spanish Potatoes

• Servings: 4 • Preparation time: 5 minutes • Cook time: 25 minutes •

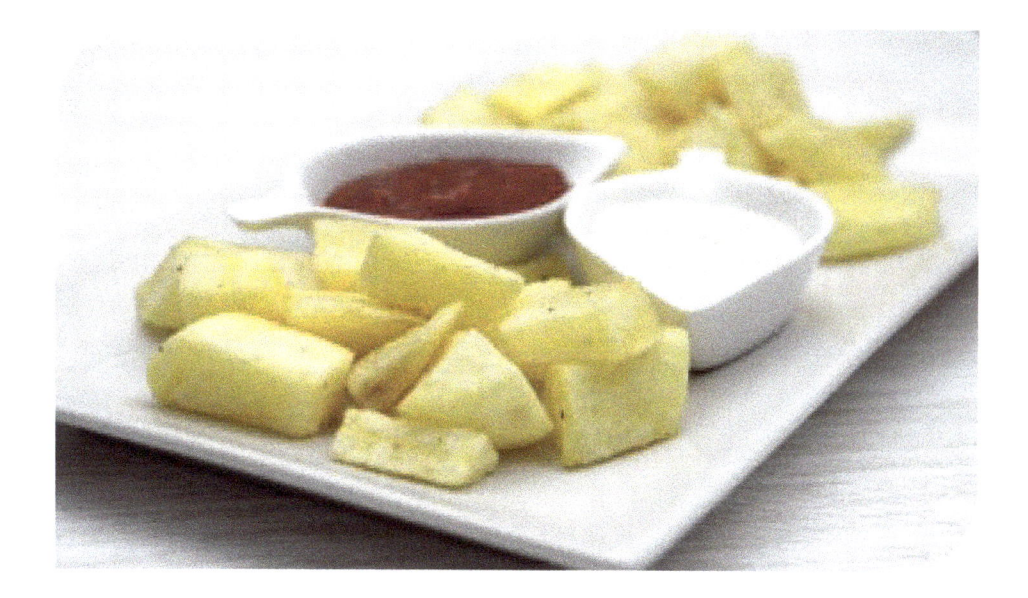

TASTY

Ingredients

- 1 pound potato
- Water
- 1 tbsp olive oil
- Salt

Steps to Cook

1. Peel and cut the potato into julienne strips approximately 0.5 cm thick

2. Prepare a bowl with very cold water, if necessary add ice. Place the cut potatoes for at least 30 minutes so that they start out in starch.

3. Dry each potato with an absorbent napkin and place in another dry bowl.

4. When they are all dry, sprinkle with oil or brush with olive oil and season with salt and whatever you like (sweet paprika, oregano, etc).

5. In this case, place in a deep fryer without oil at a temperature of 160°C for 17 minutes.

6. Set the fryer at 180°C for another 10 minutes and you're done.

Nutritional Information

- Calories: 77
- Carbohydrates: 17.47g
- Fat: 0.09g
- Protein: 2.02g
- Sugar: 0.78g
- Cholesterol: 0mg

Air Fryer Cookbook

Breaded Prawns

• Servings: 1 • Preparation time: 2 minutes • Cook time: 10 minutes •

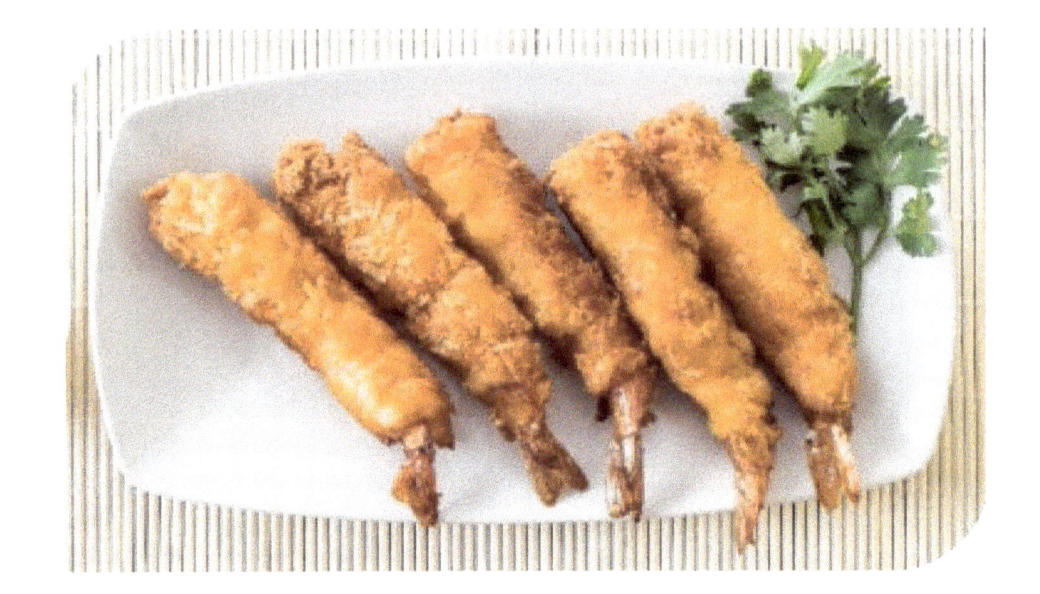

QUICK & EASY

Ingredients

- 9 raw prawns
- 1 egg
- Bread crumbs
- Condiments: salt, pepper and sweet paprika

Steps to Cook

1. If they are clean but raw and frozen, put them in water and boiled for 2 minutes.

2. Take out of the water and dry with absorbent paper.

3. Beat the egg and season to taste. Place them on a skewer stick and brush with the beaten egg. Leave in the egg until breading

4. Bread with breadcrumbs. Brush again with egg and bread again.

5. Place in the fryer strainer. Cook 5 minutes at 160ºC. Remove

6. Drizzle with fritolin or brush with oil. Place 5 more minutes in the fryer at 200ºC. Ready to enjoy them.

....

Nutritional Information

- Calories: 259
- Carbohydrates: 17.9g
- Fat: 13.7g
- Protein: 16.4g
- Sugar: 0g
- Cholesterol: 149.5mg

Pizzetas

• Servings: 4 • Preparation time: 5 minutes • Cook time: 7 minutes •

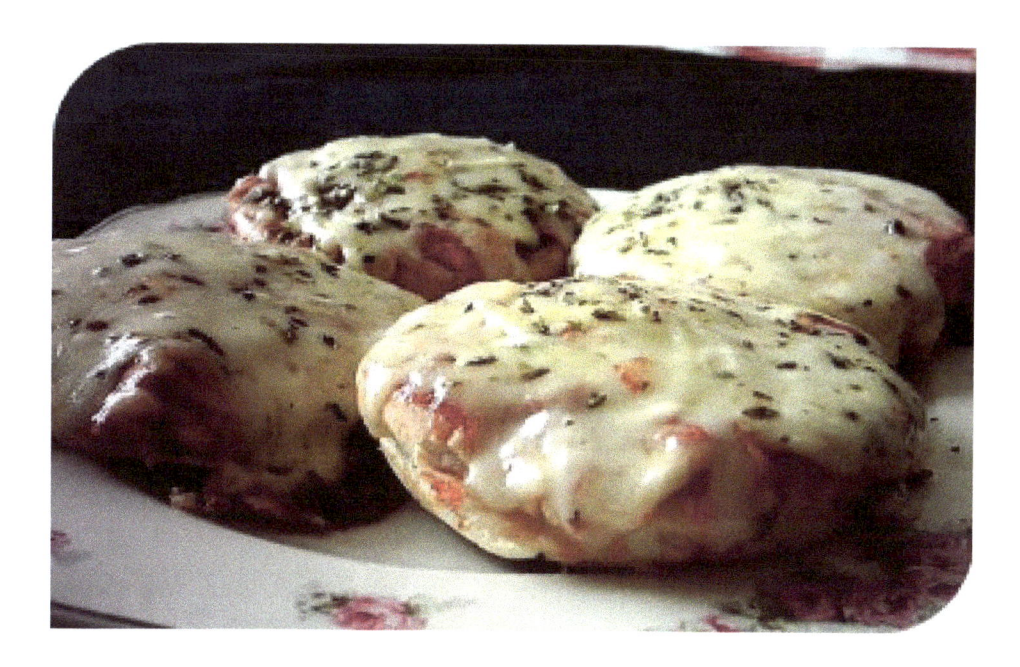

YUMMY

Ingredients

- 9 oz. flour
- ¼ oz. salt
- 1 pinch sugar
- ½ sachet instant yeast
- ½ cup warm water
- 1 splash olive oil

Sauce:

- ½ onion
- Ketchup
- Ham
- Mozzarella

Steps to Cook

1. Put the flour in a bowl with the salt, the yeast, a splash of olive oil, add the warm water and knead.

2. Leave in the bowl in a warm place so that it grows twice

3. Then divide the dough into 4 and knead into discs that go into the fryer pan without oil. Cut butter paper into discs

4. Place the dough on the paper and add the sauce, ham and cheese.

5. Put them in the pan one by one about 7 minutes at 150ºC.

Nutritional Information

- Calories: 232
- Carbohydrates: 30.27g
- Fat: 8.3g
- Protein: 8.54g
- Sugar: 1.3g
- Cholesterol: 13mg

Air Fryer Cookbook

Wings with fine herbs

• Servings: 2 • Preparation time: 1h 2 minutes • Cook time: 10 minutes •

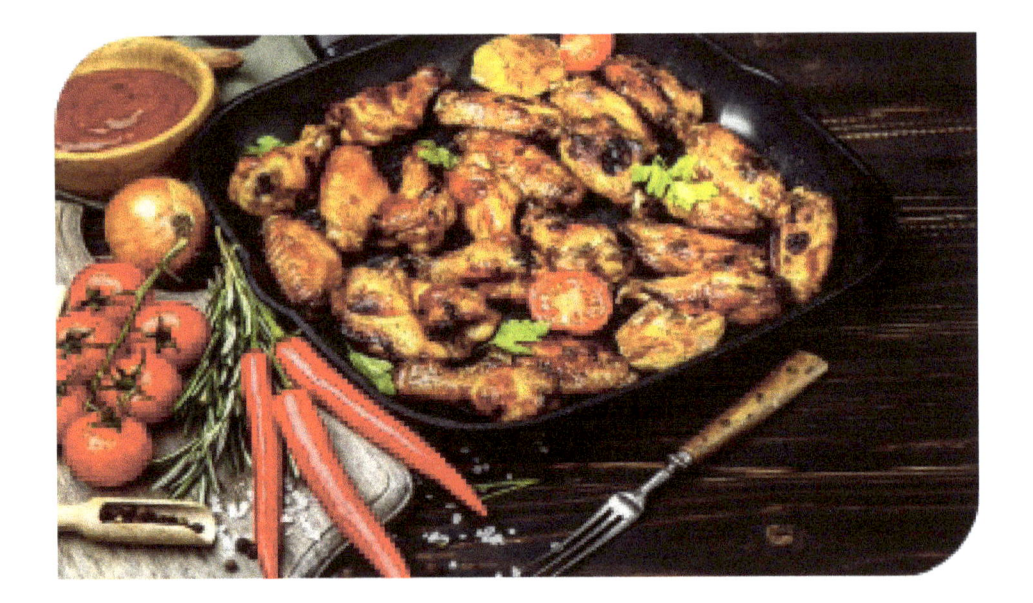

GORGEOUS

Ingredients

- 2 lbs wings
- 1 sachet of magui with fine herbs
- Chilli
- Tomatoes
- The juice of a lemon
- Salt

Steps to Cook

1. Marinate the wings with the spices and the lemon, leave 1 hour.

2. Set the fryer to preheat for about 10 minutes, fry menu temperature 200ºC.

3. Put the wings in the bowl and go around from time to time, remove and serve.

Nutritional Information

- Calories: 180
- Carbohydrates: 2g
- Fat: 9g
- Protein: 22g
- Sugar: 1g
- Cholesterol: 240mg

Chopped Bondiola

• Servings: 4 • Preparation time: 5 minutes • Cook time: 20 minutes •

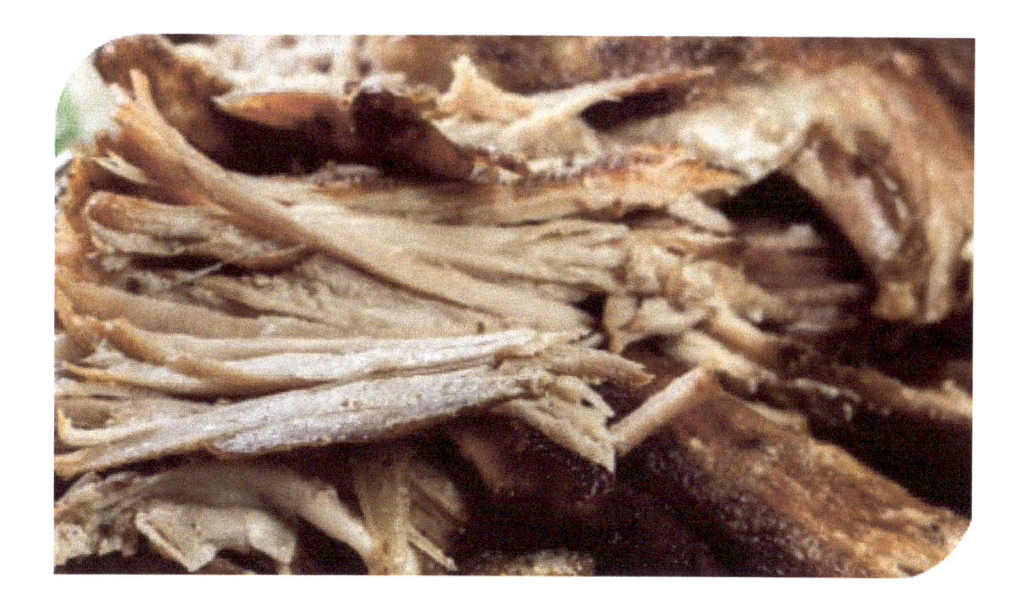

LIGHTLY BREADED

Ingredients

- 2 lbs bondiola chunks
- Bread crumbs
- 2 eggs
- Seasoning to taste

Steps to Cook

1. Cut the bondiola into small pieces, seasonings to taste.

2. Beat the eggs.

3. Pass the bondiola seasoned with beaten egg and then with breadcrumbs.

4. Then put in the air fryer for 20 minutes at 150ºC, half time turn and ready bondiola sandwiches.

Nutritional Information

- Calories: 265
- Carbohydrates: 0g
- Fat: 20.36g
- Protein: 19.14g
- Sugar: 0g
- Cholesterol: 146mg

Zucchini sticks

• Servings: 1 • Preparation time: 30 minutes • Cook time: 20 minutes •

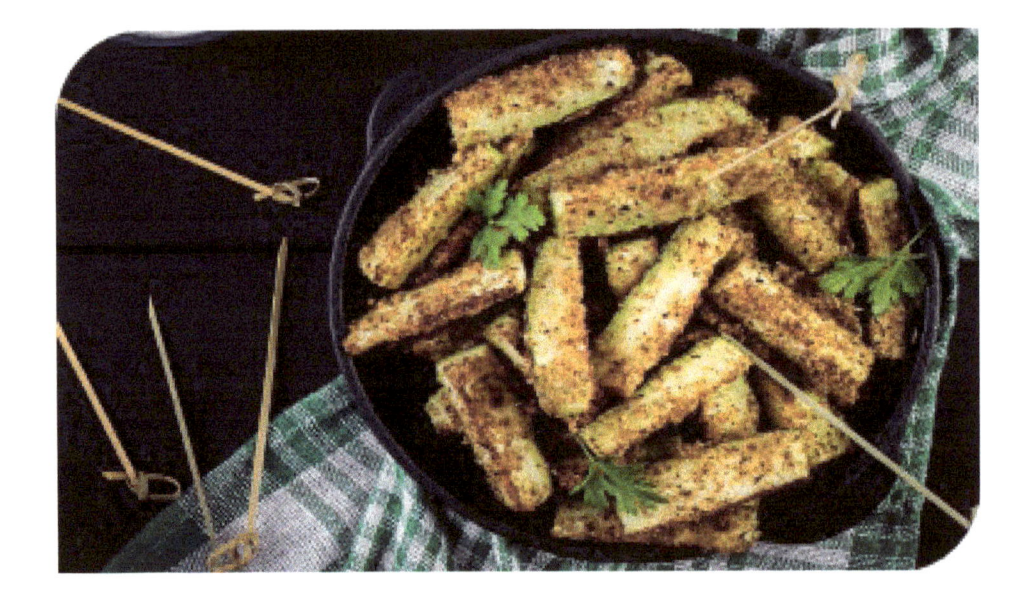

MOUTHWATERING

Ingredients

- 1 zucchini
- 2 eggs
- 1 cup flour
- 1 lemon
- 1 cup grated cheese and breadcrumbs

Steps to Cook

1. Cut the zucchini into sticks.

2. Have a bowl with flour, another with the seasoned eggs and a last one with the lemon zest, grated cheese and breadcrumbs all together and mixed.

3. Pass all the zucchinis by flour, then by the eggs and finally by the mixture of lemon, cheese and breadcrumbs.

4. Take to deep fryer without oil or preheated for approximately 20 minutes at 180ºC and ready!

....

Nutritional Information

- Calories: 427
- Carbohydrates: 41g
- Fat: 24g
- Protein: 11.7g
- Sugar: 9g
- Cholesterol: 111mg

Pumpkin Croquettes

• Servings: 4 • Preparation time: 5 minutes • Cook time: 23 minutes •

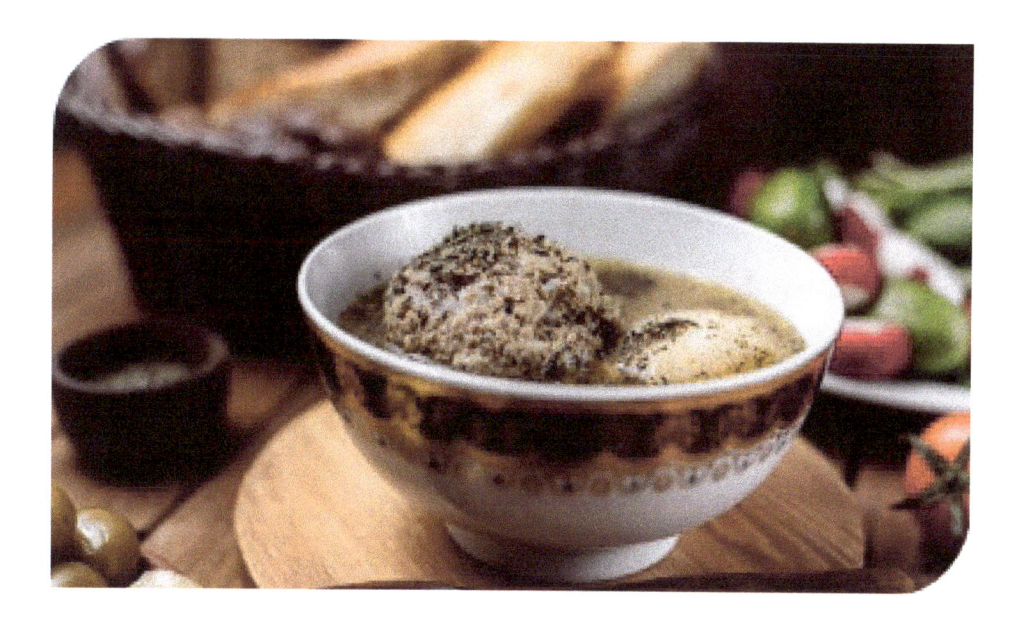

FRUITY

Ingredients

- Pumpkin puree
- 1 onion
- 1 tbsp or 2 tbsp grated cheese
- Eggs
- Bread crumbs
- Light cheese

Steps to Cook

1. Make pumpkin puree.

2. Sauté small cut onion, cook it in water and they are very good.

3. Mix in a bowl, the pumpkin, grated cheese, onion, salt, pepper and nutmeg.

4. Assemble the croquettes, and put cheese, in the middle, go through breadcrumbs, beaten egg and breadcrumbs.

5. Put vegetable spray, 200ºC and 20 minutes and ready.

Nutritional Information

- Calories: 81
- Carbohydrates: 8g
- Fat: 4g
- Protein: 1g
- Sugar: 0g
- Cholesterol: 300mg

Air Fryer Cookbook

Fritters Chard

• Servings: 4 • Preparation time: 5minutes • Cook time: 15 minutes •

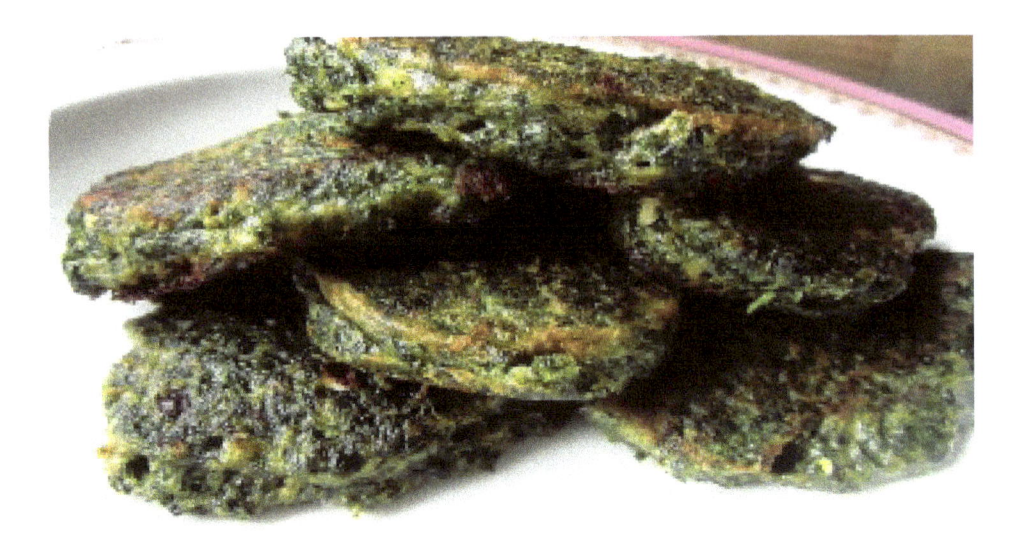

TOASTED

Ingredients

- 3 ½ oz. whole wheat flour
- 3 eggs
- 1 chard bouquet
- 5 tbsp mix seeds
- 1 tbsp baking powder
- Salt
- Pepper
- 2 tbsp olive oil
- 1 cup milk

Steps to Cook

1. Wash the chard.

2. Cook the chard for a minute, then proceed to cut it finely.

3. In a bowl place the three eggs with the milk and the seed and beat.

4. Place the cut chard in the bowl, then gradually add the flour, baking powder and oil.

5. Turn on your fryer, set it to about 180°C, and wait a few minutes for it to heat up.

6. With the fritolin, rub the basket and place the previously prepared mixture with a spoon.

7. After 15 minutes turn around so that it is golden on the other side.

Nutritional Information

- Calories: 64
- Carbohydrates: 4.8g
- Fat: 4.2g
- Protein: 2g
- Sugar: 0.4g
- Cholesterol: 24mg

Grilled Squid

• Servings:1 • Preparation time: 5 minutes • Cook time: 10 minutes •

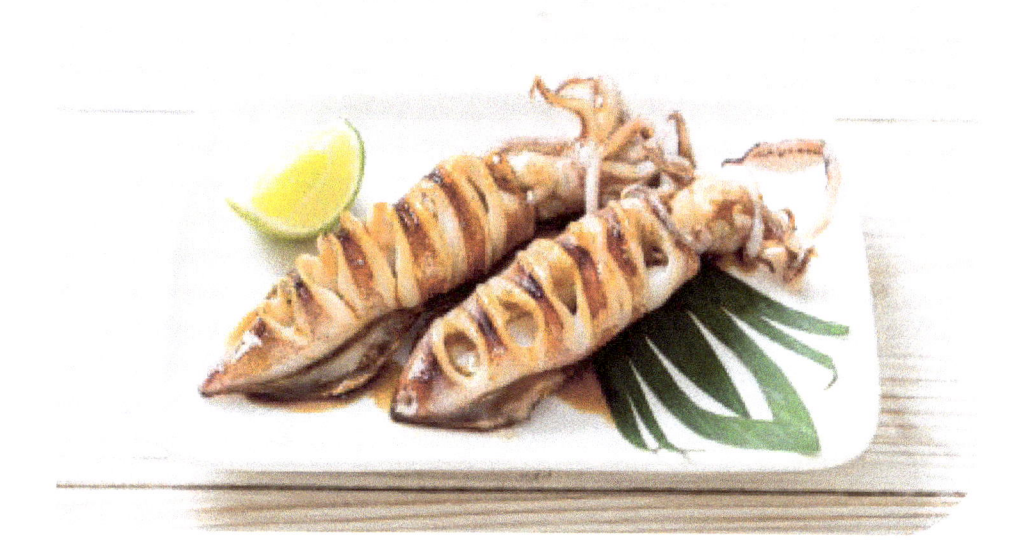

RICH

Ingredients

- 6 medium squid
- Salt
- 2 tbsp extra virgin olive oil
- 1 clove garlic
- Parsley

Steps to Cook

1. Clean the squid and season.

2. Put 1 tablespoon of oil and with our hands we smear well on all sides.

3. Put them in the fryer basket and set 200°C 10 minutes and ready.

4. In a bowl put the other tablespoon of oil with the minced garlic and a little parsley, stir and integrate everything well.

5. Pour over the oil with the garlic and eat.

Nutritional Information

- Calories: 290
- Carbohydrates: 12g
- Fat: 3g
- Protein: 48g
- Sugar: 0g
- Cholesterol: 300mg

Iberian Prey Fillets

• Servings: 6 • Preparation time: 5 minutes • Cook time: 10 minutes •

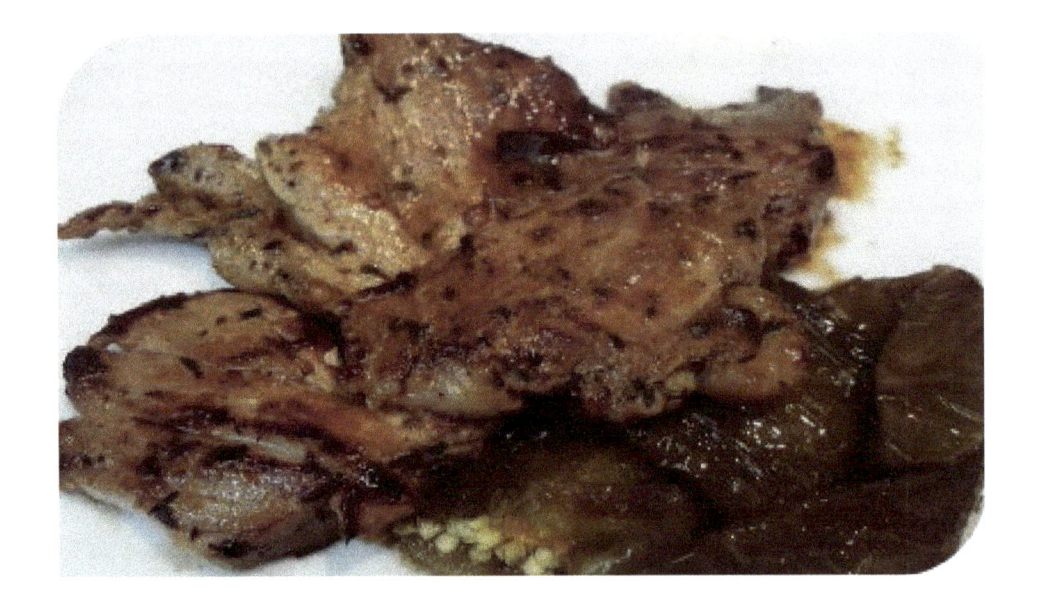

HEALTHY

Ingredients

- 4 Iberian pork fillets
- 1 Tbsp olive oil
- 1 pinch sweet paprika
- Salt

Steps to Cook

1. Put the seasoned fillets in the basket and brush with the oil, program 200ºC for 10 minutes.

2. Serve together with the potatoes a super light, healthy and rich dinner.

Nutritional Information

- Calories: 216
- Carbohydrates: 0g
- Fat: 14g
- Protein: 21.1g
- Sugar: 0g
- Cholesterol: 300mg

Milanesas of stuffed stalks

• Servings: 2 • Preparation time: 5 minutes • Cook time: 15 minutes •

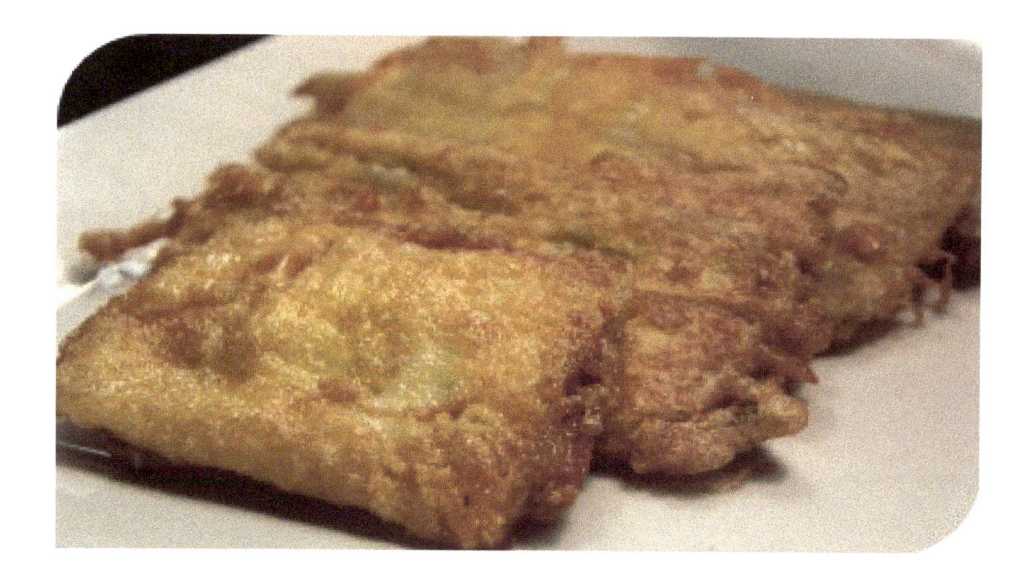

QUICK

Ingredients

- Boiled broad stalks
- Quartirolo cheese
- Cooked shoulder
- Egg
- Flour to coat
- Bread crumbs
- Condiments to taste
- 1 sachet bacon flavor powder
- Oil for frying or deep fryer without oil

Steps to Cook

1. Put the leaves on the counter even number, with the palette and cheese make a roll. Put the same on a stalk.

2. Cover with the other sheet. As if you were making a sandwich. Go through flour. Reserve.

3. Beat the egg with the seasonings and flavoring combine everything very well. Pass the reserved stalks for egg and breadcrumbs.

4. Put in the air fryer at 240ºC for 15 minutes.

Nutritional Information

- Calories: 8
- Carbohydrates: 1g
- Fat: 0g
- Protein: 1g
- Sugar: 0g
- Cholesterol: 300mg

Air Fryer Cookbook

Potatoes Cheese And Bacon

• Servings: 4 • Preparation time: 10 minutes • Cook time: 5 minutes •

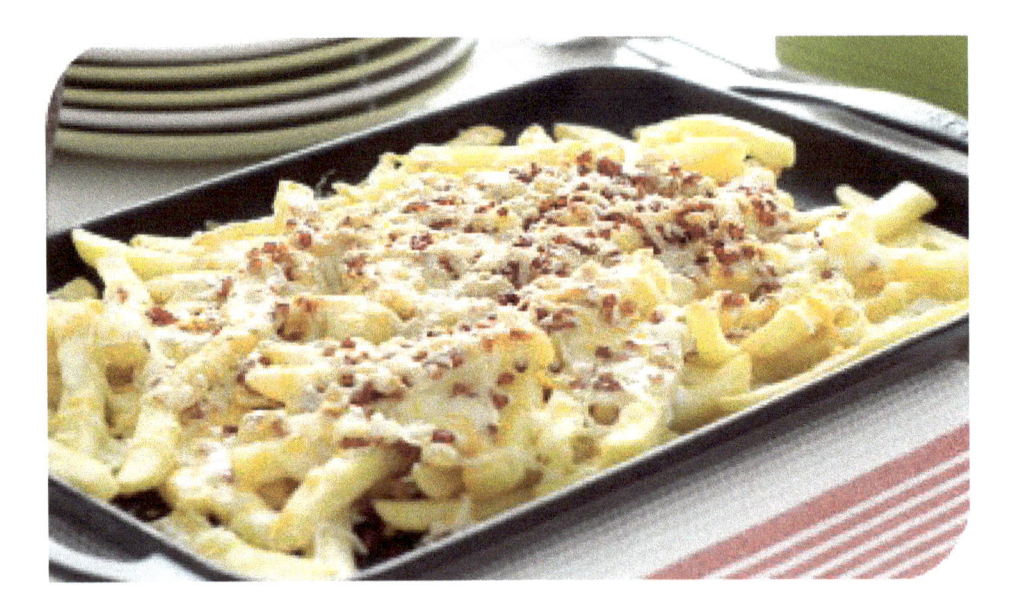

APPETIZING

Ingredients

- 1 pound potato chips from the oven or deep fryer
- 1 Package 4 grated cheeses
- 1 package bacon
- Ranchera Sauce

Steps to Cook

1. Firstly, gather the ingredients.

2. Put the fried potatoes in a bowl or container to make them in a deep fryer

3. Make the bacon in a separate pan

4. Mix the fried potatoes and the bacon, also add the cheese you want and leave it in the air fryer at 180ºC for about 5 minutes until the cheese melts

Nutritional Information

- Calories: 336
- Carbohydrates: 69.9g
- Fat: 18.5g
- Protein: 0g
- Sugar: 9g
- Cholesterol: 82mg

Goat Cheese Salad

• Servings: 1 • Preparation time: 5 minutes • Cook time: 5 minutes •

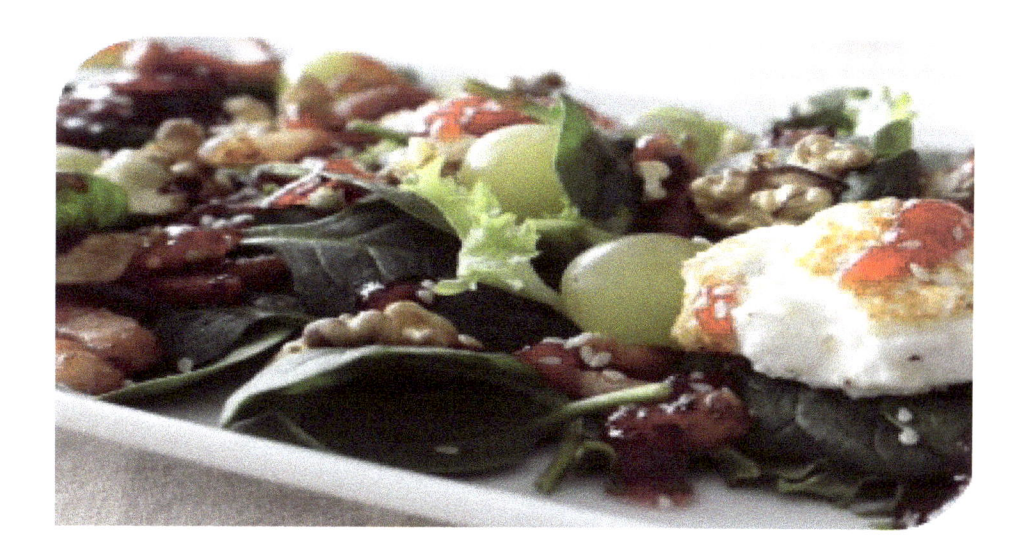

DELICIOUS

Ingredients

- 1 lettuce head
- 1 pack Super Smoked Salmon
- 1 anchovy in oil
- Salt
- 1 bottle Balsamic oil of Modena
- 1 roll of goat cheese
- 1 egg
- bread crumbs

Steps to Cook

1. Cut the goat cheese, into portions and pass it through egg and breadcrumbs

2. Cut the bud in 4 parts across the width and put at the base of the plate with a pinch of salt, then a little Smoked Salmon, then the Goat cheese, which before you will have gone through the air fryer at 190°C for 5 minutes. Put half of 1 anchovy and put in Modern Balsamic Oil.

3. Put some combined nuts from the super that are already prepared.

Nutritional Information

- Calories: 621
- Carbohydrates: 40g
- Fat: 50g
- Protein: 8g
- Sugar: 32g
- Cholesterol: 17mg

Air Fryer Cookbook

Chorizo Stuffings

• Servings: 4 • Preparation time: 5 minutes • Cook time: 20 minutes •

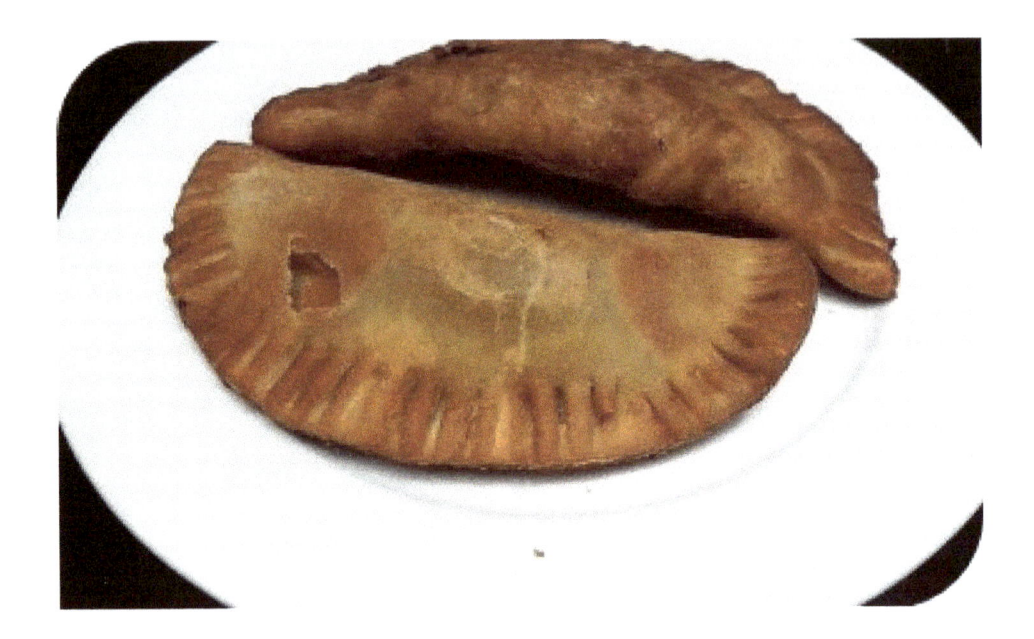

LOVELY

Ingredients

- 4 ½ oz. chorizo in small tacos
- 1 chopped onion
- ¼ red bell pepper cut into tiny strips
- 2 tbsp of parsley
- ½ lb of shortcrust pastry.

Steps to Cook

1. In the first place fry all these ingredients (without oil) over a low heat since it will be the sausage itself that will expel the fat.

2. Secondly, when the pepper is tender, remove it from the heat and pre-heat it in the fryer at 200ºC.

3. With a mold cut the shortcrust pastry in a circle, place a tablespoon of the chorizo mixture in each of the circles and join the edges with a fork so that they are well glued. Finally, put the empanadas in the fryer basket, adjust the timer to 20 minutes and bake to brown.

Nutritional Information

- Calories: 757
- Carbohydrates: 36g
- Fat: 33g
- Protein: 73g
- Sugar: 4g
- Cholesterol: 300mg

Brazilian Chicken Thighs

• Servings: 2 • Preparation time: 5 minutes • Cook time: 25 minutes •

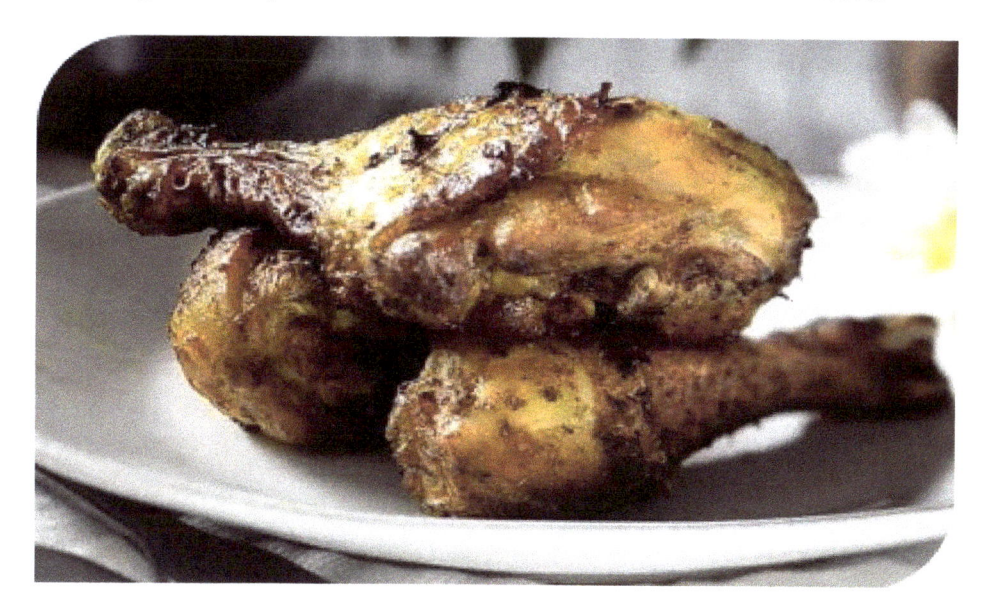

FLAVORSOME

Ingredients

- 1 tsp of cumin seeds
- 1 tsp dried oregano
- 1 tsp of dried parsley
- 1 tsp ground turmeric
- ½ tsp coriander seeds
- 1 tsp of kosher salt
- ½ tsp black peppercorns
- ½ tsp of pepper
- ¼ cup fresh lime juice
- 2 tsp of olive oil
- 1 ½ pounds chicken

Steps to Cook

1. In a clean coffee grinder or spice mill, combine cumin, oregano, parsley, turmeric, coriander seeds, salt, peppercorns, and cayenne pepper. Process until finely ground

2. In a small bowl, combine the ground spices with lemon juice and oil. Place the chicken in a zippered bag. Add marinade, seal and massage until chicken is well coated. Marinate at room temperature for 30 minutes or in the refrigerator for up to 24 hours.

3. When it is ready to cook, place skin-side up in the fryer basket. Adjust the air fryer to 400°C for 20-25 minutes, turning the legs halfway through the cooking time. Use a meat thermometer to make sure the chicken has reached an internal temperature of 165 C.

Nutritional Information

- Calories: 255
- Carbohydrates: 3g
- Fat: 15g
- Protein: 20g
- Sugar: 1g
- Cholesterol: 105mg

Air Fryer Cookbook

Lemon Chicken Recipe

• Servings: 4 • Preparation time: 5 minutes • Cook time: 20 minutes •

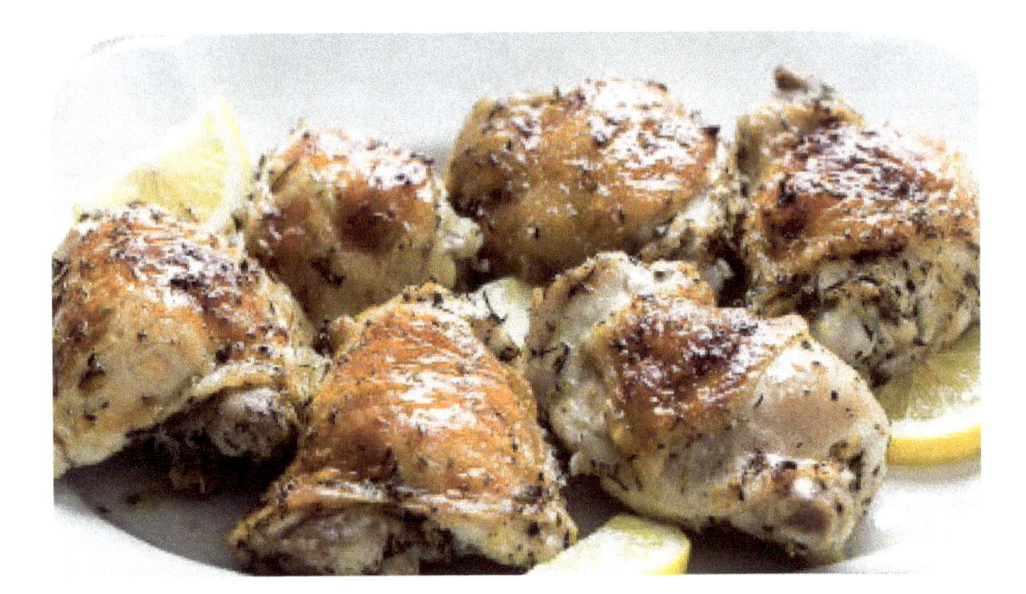

LEMONADE

Ingredients

- 6 chicken
- 2 tbsp of olive oil
- 2 tbsp of lemon juice
- 1 tbsp of Italian herb seasoning mix
- 1 tsp Celtic sea salt
- 1 tsp freshly ground pepper
- 1 lemon, thinly sliced

Steps to Cook

1. Add all ingredients except sliced lemon to bowl or bag, stir to coat chicken. Let marinate for 30 minutes overnight. Remove chicken and allow excess oil to drip.

2. Arrange the chicken thighs and lemon slices in the fryer basket, being careful not to push the chicken thighs too close to each other.

3. Set the fryer to 350ºC and cook for 10 minutes.

4. Remove the basket from the fryer and turn the chicken thighs over to the other side.

5. Cook again at 350ºC for another 10 minutes.

6. Chicken will be crispy, with clear juices and will reach 165ºC internal temperature when verified with a digital thermometer inserted into the thickest part of the thigh.

Nutritional Information

- Calories: 325
- Carbohydrates: 2g
- Fat: 23g
- Protein: 31g
- Sugar: 0g
- Cholesterol: 166mg

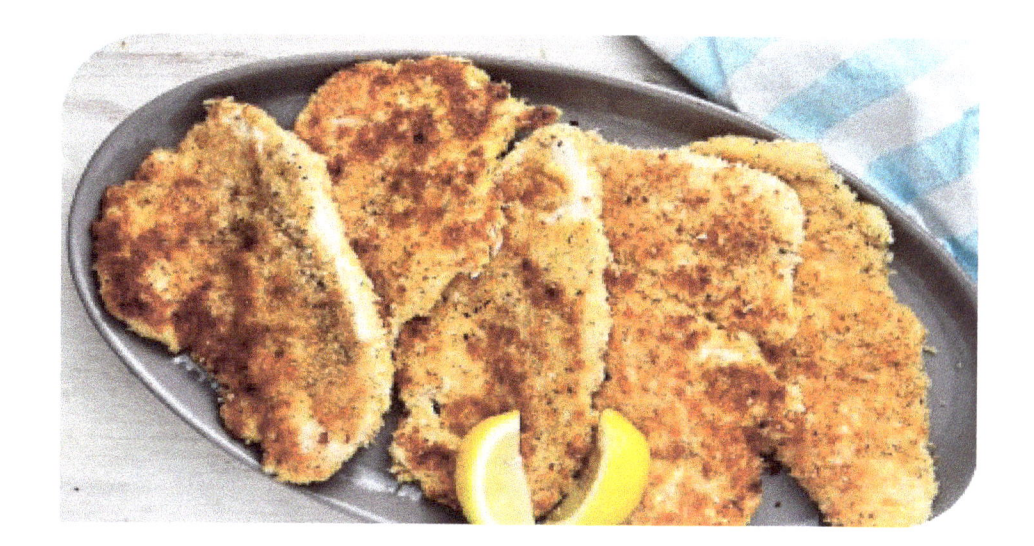

CRUNCHY

Parmesan Chicken

• Servings: 2 • Preparation time: 1 minutes • Cook time: 12 minutes •

Ingredients

- 1 ½ oz. Italian-style breadcrumbs
- ½ oz. parmesan cheese
- 2 chicken breasts
- 2 oz. all-purpose flour
- 2 eggs, beaten
- Non-stick spray oil
- 2 slices of mozzarella cheese
- Marinara sauce, to serve
- 2 sprigs of parsley, freshly chopped, for garnish

Steps to Cook

1. Select Preheat, in the air fryer adjust the temperature to 180°C and press Start/Pause.

2. Mix the breadcrumbs and Parmesan cheese in a bowl.

3. Pass each chicken breast through the flour, then dip them in the beaten eggs and, finally, in the crumb mixture.

4. Drizzle the inside of the preheated air fryer baskets with cooking oil and place the chicken breasts inside, also sprinkling the top of the chicken.

5. Cook the chicken breasts at 180°C for 12 minutes.

6. Put 1 slice of mozzarella cheese on each breast when 2 minutes are left on the timer.

7. Serve with marinara sauce and garnish with freshly chopped parsley.

Nutritional Information

- Calories: 320
- Carbohydrates: 20g
- Fat: 19g
- Protein: 17g
- Sugar: 3g
- Cholesterol: 55mg

Air Fryer Cookbook

Eggplant Escalope

• Servings: 2 • Preparation time: 8 minutes • Cook time: 8 minutes •

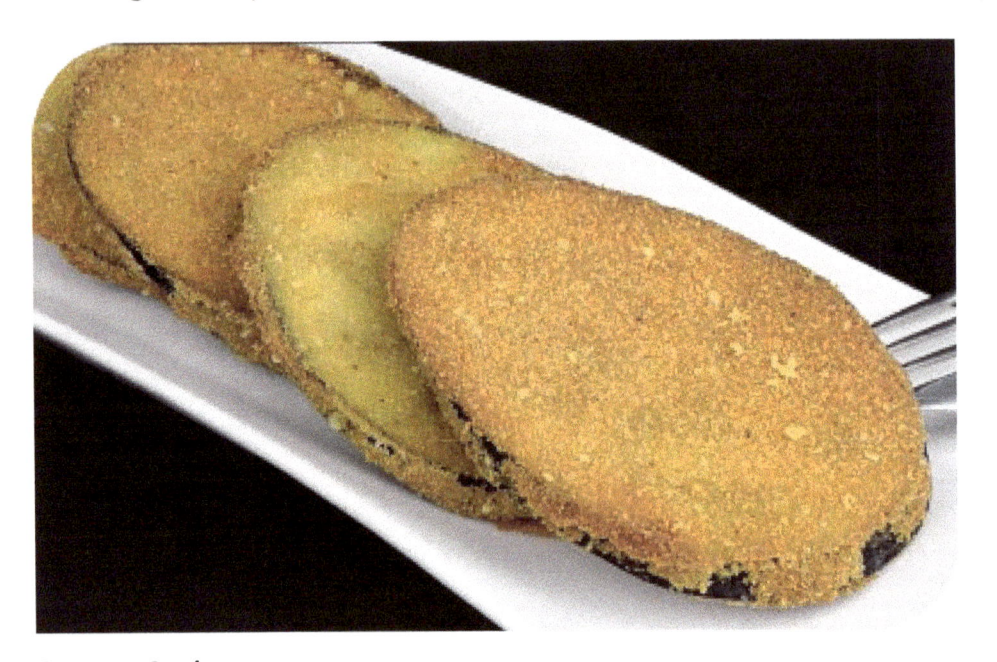

TOASTED

Ingredients

- 1 egg, beaten
- 3 tsp milk
- 4 oz. Italian-style breadcrumbs
- ½ tsp of salt
- ¼ tsp black pepper
- 1 Japanese eggplant, cut into 13 mm thick slices
- 2 oz. all-purpose flour
- Olive oil, for brushing

Steps to Cook

1. Beat the egg and milk in a shallow bowl. Combine the breadcrumbs, salt, and pepper on a separate plate.

2. Cut the eggplant into 13mm thick slices.

3. Cover the eggplant slices with flour, then dip them in egg and stir in breadcrumbs. Dip them in egg and breadcrumbs again.

4. Select Preheat on the air fryer and press Start/Pause.

5. Brush each side of the eggplant slices with olive oil.

6. Place the breaded eggplant in the preheated air fryer in a single layer and cook at 205°C for 8 minutes. You may have to work in batches.

7. Flip the eggplant halfway through cooking.

Nutritional Information

- Calories: 55
- Carbohydrates: 10.1g
- Fat: 1g
- Protein: 2.4g
- Sugar: 2.6g
- Cholesterol: 21.3mg

Crispy Tofu

• Servings: 2 • Preparation time: 15 minutes • Cook time: 18minutes •

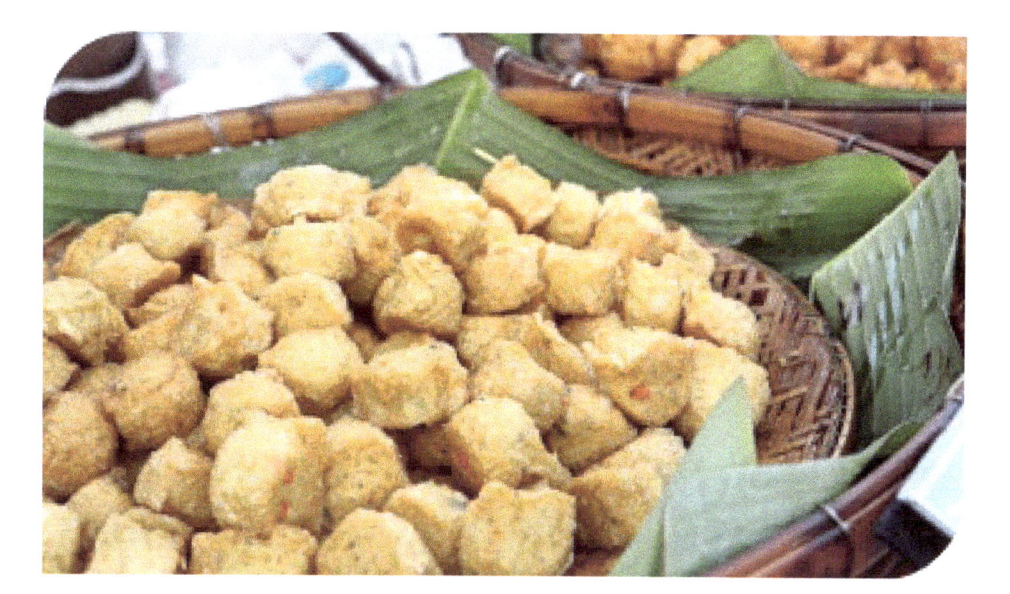

CRISPY

Ingredients

- ½ lb firm tofu, cut into 25mm cubes
- 6 tsp soy sauce
- 2 tsp of rice vinegar
- 2 tsp sesame oil
- 1 ½ oz. cornstarch

Steps to Cook

1. Wash the carrots very well and remove the ends.

2. Cut the carrots into very thin slices, either using a mandolin or with a food processor.

3. Add the oil and with clean hands, spread it over all the carrots. Put the carrot slices in the basket of your air fryer and program it at 165ºC for 20-25 minutes, depending on the amount of carrots you make.

4. Every 5-7 minutes open the basket and shake it vigorously so that they are removed, and put the basket back inside so that they continue to be made. Watch from the 15th minute that they do not burn, since it depends on the amount you do can be done before. Take out the carrots, put some salt on them and ready.

Nutritional Information

- Calories: 127
- Carbohydrates: 13.7g
- Fat: 5.9g
- Protein: 5.7g
- Sugar: 0.1g
- Cholesterol: 0mg

Air Fryer Cookbook

Salmon with Butter and Lemon

• Servings: 2 • Preparation time: 3 minutes • Cook time: 8 minutes •

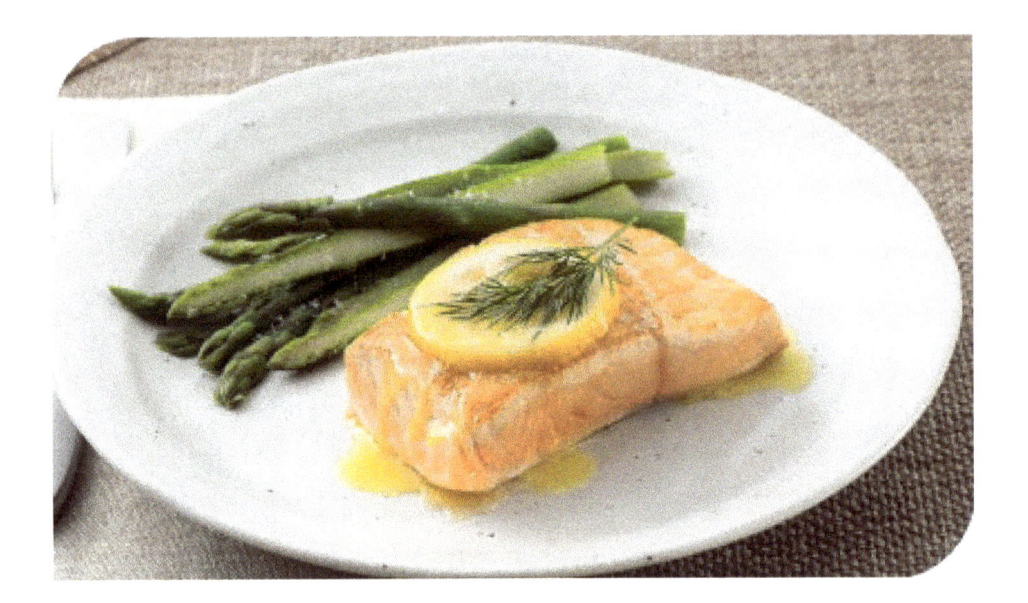

YUMMY

Ingredients

- 2 salmon fillets (6 oz)
- Salt and pepper to taste
- Non-stick spray oil
- 1 oz. of butter
- 6 tsp of fresh lemon juice
- 1 garlic clove, grated
- 1 tsp Worcestershire sauce

Steps to Cook

1. Season the salmon to taste with salt and pepper.

2. Select Preheat, in the air fryer adjust the temperature to 175°C and press Start/Pause.

3. Spray baskets in preheated air fryer with cooking spray and place fish inside.

4. Select Seafood and press Start/Pause.

5. Combine butter, lemon juice, garlic, and Worcestershire sauce in small saucepan and simmer, about 1 minute.

6. Serve the salmon fillets with beans and top with the lemon butter sauce.

Nutritional Information

- Calories: 505
- Carbohydrates: 1.4g
- Fat: 35g
- Protein: 43g
- Sugar: 0.1g
- Cholesterol: 152mg

Teriyaki Salmon

• Servings: 2 • Preparation time: 10 minutes • Cook time: 8 minutes •

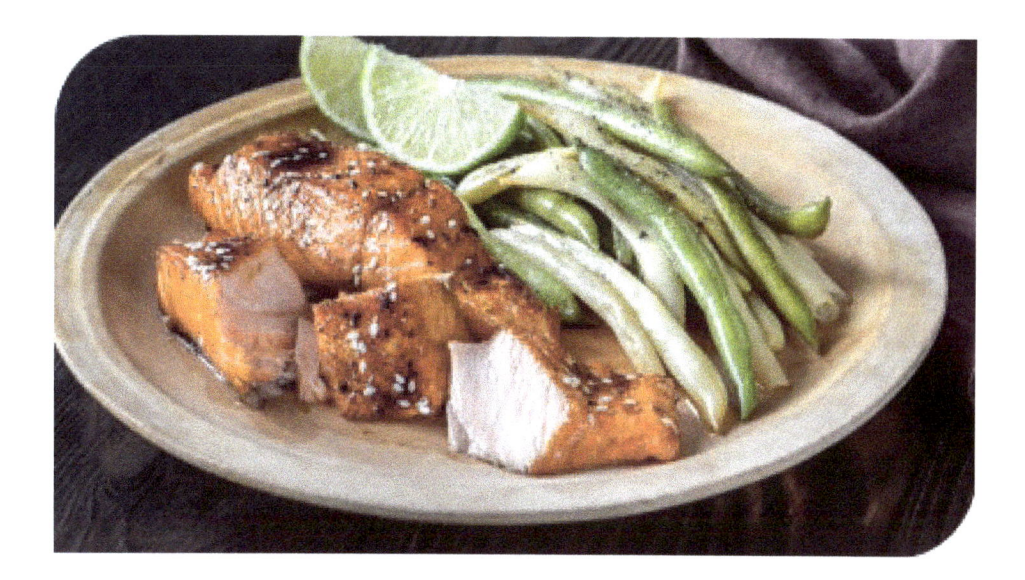

Ingredients

Teriyaki sauce:

- ½ cup soy sauce
- ¼ cup of sugar
- ¼ tsp of grated ginger
- 1 garlic clove, crushed
- ¼ cup orange juice

Salmon:

- 2 salmon fillets (5 oz)
- 4 tsp of vegetable oil
- Salt and white pepper, to taste

Steps to Cook

1. Combine all the ingredients for the teriyaki sauce in a small saucepan. Bring the sauce to a boil, cut it in half, then let it cool.

2. Select Preheat, in the air fryer adjust the temperature to 175°C and press Start/Pause.

3. Cover the salmon with oil and season with salt and white pepper. Place the salmon in the preheated air fryer, facing down. Select Seafood, set to 8 minutes, and press Start/Pause.

4. Remove the salmon from the fryer when done. Let stand 5 minutes, then glaze with teriyaki sauce.

5. Serve with beans.

Nutritional Information

- Calories: 233
- Carbohydrates: 11.3g
- Fat: 5.5g
- Protein: 33.6g
- Sugar: 7.5g
- Cholesterol: 83mg

Tasty Tuna Chipotle

• Servings: 2 • Preparation time: 5 minutes • Cook time: 40 minutes •

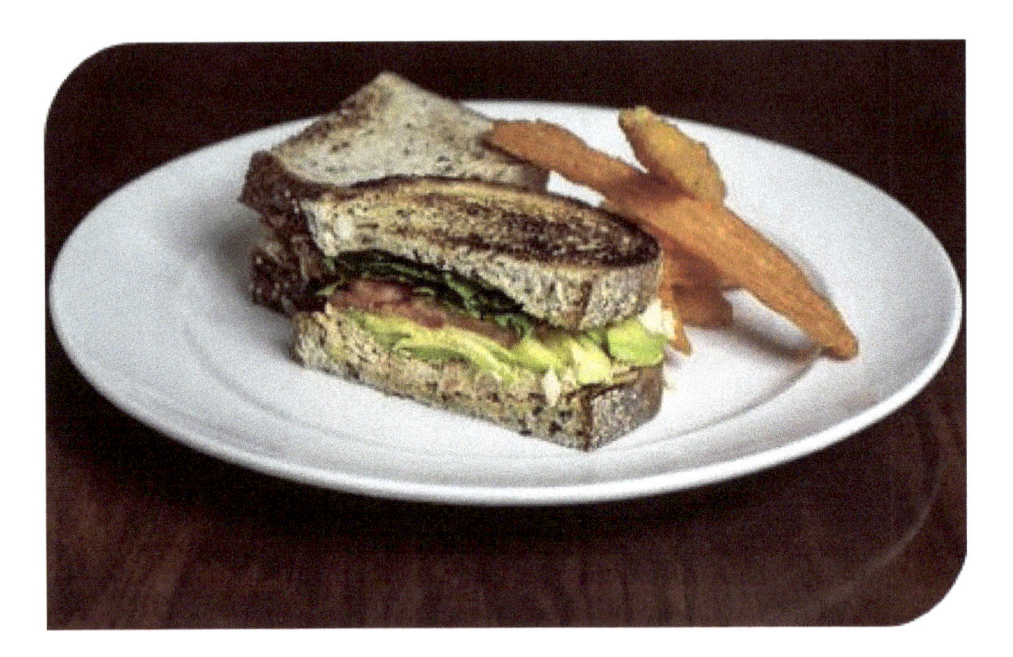

TASTY

Ingredients

- 1 can tuna
- 1 ½ oz. chipotle sauce
- 4 slices of white bread
- 2 slices of pepper jack cheese

Steps to Cook

1. Select Preheat, in the air fryer adjust the temperature to 160°C and press Start/Pause.

2. Mix the tuna and chipotle until combined.

3. Spread half of the chipotle tuna mixture on each of the 2 slices of bread.

4. Add a slice of pepper jack cheese to each and close with the remaining 2 slices of bread, making 2 sandwiches.

5. Place the sandwiches in the preheated air fryer.

6. Select Pan, set the time to 8 minutes and press Start/Pause.

7. Cut diagonally and serve.

Nutritional Information

- Calories: 70
- Carbohydrates: 1g
- Fat: 0.5g
- Protein: 15g
- Sugar: 0g
- Cholesterol: 20mg

Cajun Catfish

• Servings: 2 • Preparation time: 3 minutes • Cook time: 7 minutes •

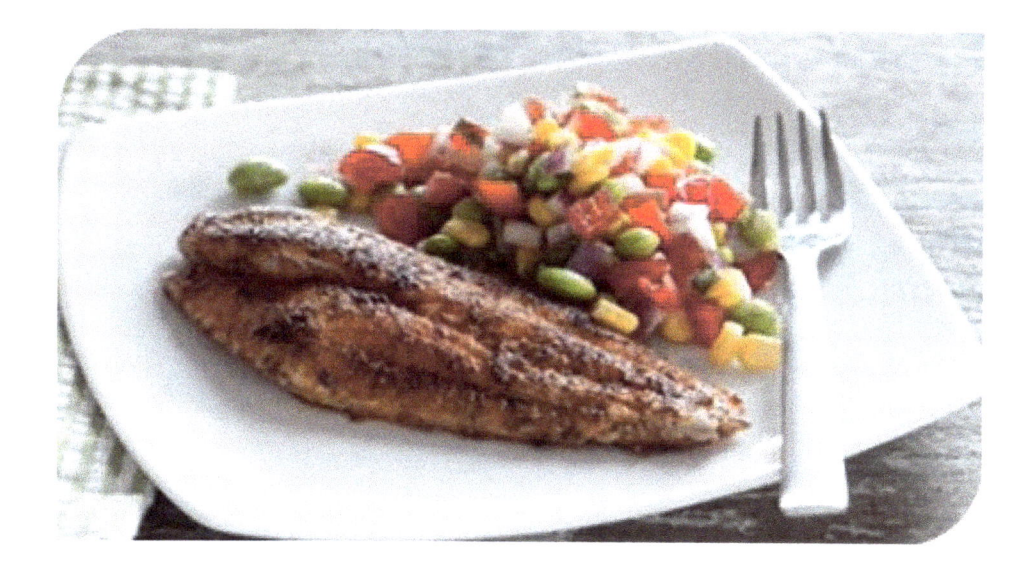

MOUTH WATERING

Ingredients

- 1 tsp paprika
- ½ tsp garlic powder
- ½ tsp onion powder
- ½ tsp dried ground thyme
- 1/3 tsp of ground black pepper
- 1 g of cayenne pepper
- 1/3 tsp dried basil
- ¼ tsp dried oregano
- 2 catfish fillets (6 oz)
- Non-stick spray oil

Steps to Cook

1. Select Preheat, in the air fryer adjust the temperature to 175°C and press Start/Pause.

2. Mix all the seasonings in a bowl.

3. Coat the fish liberally on each side with the dressing mixture.

4. Spray each side of the fish with cooking spray and place it in the preheated air fryer.

5. Select Seafood and press Start/Pause.

6. Remove carefully when you finish cooking and serve on semolina.

Nutritional Information

- Calories: 301
- Carbohydrates: 0g
- Fat: 18g
- Protein: 36g
- Sugar: 0g
- Cholesterol: 190mg

Air Fryer Cookbook

Katsu Pig

• Servings: 2 • Preparation time: 10 minutes • Cook time: 14 minutes •

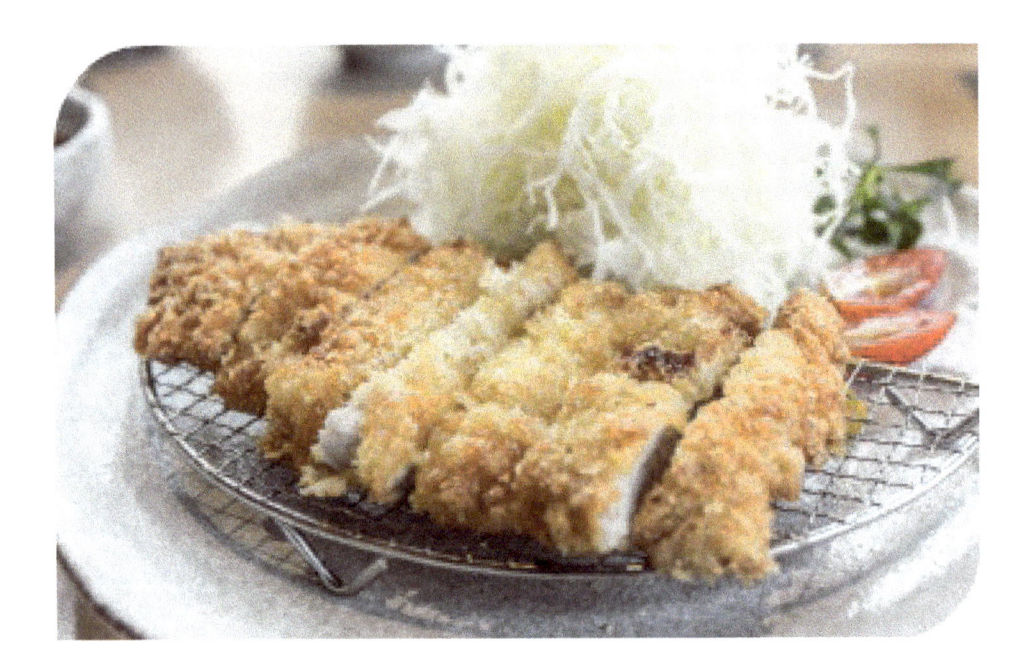

TOOTHSOME

Ingredients

- 6 oz. pork chops, boneless
- 2 oz. breadcrumbs
- ½ tsp garlic powder
- 1/3 tsp onion powder
- 1 tsp of salt
- ¼ tsp of white pepper
- 2 oz. all-purpose flour
- 2 eggs, smoothies
- Non-stick spray oil

Steps to Cook

1. Place the pork chops in an airtight bag or cover them with plastic wrap. Crush the pork with a rolling pin or meat hammer until it is 13 mm thick.

2. Combine the crumbs and seasonings in a bowl. Leave aside. Pass each pork chop through the flour, then soak them in the beaten eggs and finally pass them through the crumb mixture.

3. Select Preheat, in the air fryer adjust the temperature to 180°C and press Start/Pause. Drizzle the pork chops on each side with cooking oil and place in the preheated air fryer. Cook pork chops at 180°C for 4 minutes. Remove them from the air fryer when you're done and let them sit for 5 minutes. Cut them into pieces and serve.

Nutritional Information

- Calories: 312
- Carbohydrates: 24g
- Fat: 10g
- Protein: 29g
- Sugar: 2g
- Cholesterol: 133mg

Pork Chops

• Servings: 2 • Preparation time: 5 minutes • Cook time: 10 minutes •

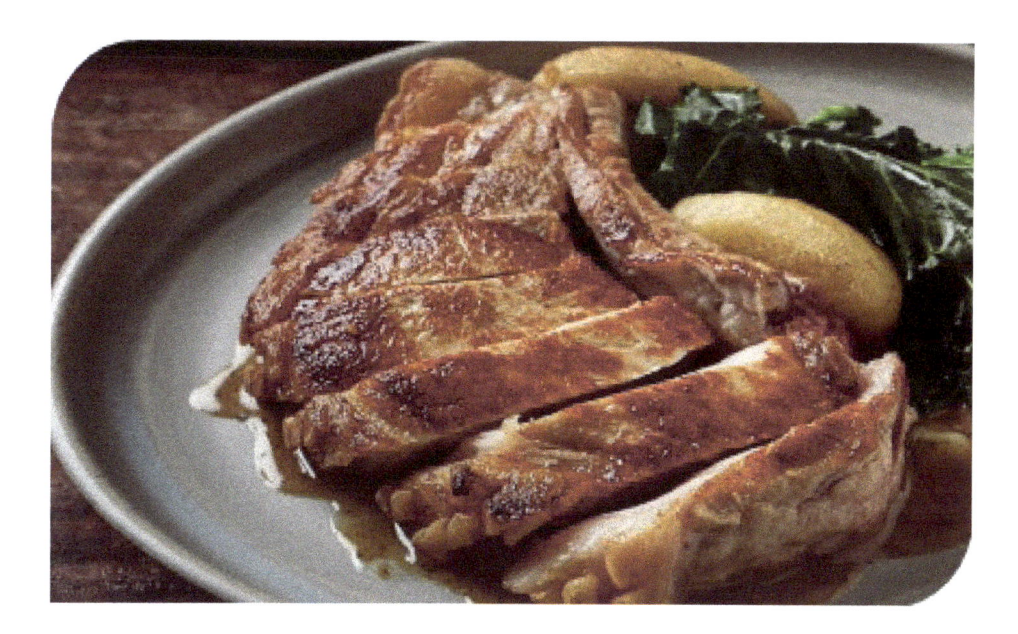

AMAZINGLY DELICIOUS

Ingredients

- 6 oz. boneless pork chops
- 3 tsp of vegetable oil
- 1 oz. brown sugar,
- 1 ½ tsp paprika
- ½ tsp of ground mustard
- ½ tsp freshly ground black pepper
- 1 tsp onion powder
- ½ tsp garlic powder
- Salt and pepper

Steps to Cook

1. Select Preheat, on the air fryer and press Start/Pause.
2. Cover the pork chops with oil.
3. Combine all the spices and season the pork chops abundantly, almost as if you were breading them.
4. Place the pork chops in the preheated air fryer.
5. Select Fillet, set the time to 10 minutes and press Start/Pause.
6. Remove the pork chops when you're done cooking, let them steep for 5 minutes and serve.

Nutritional Information

- Calories: 220
- Carbohydrates: 0g
- Fat: 14g
- Protein: 23.1g
- Sugar: 0g
- Cholesterol: 75mg

Air Fryer Cookbook

Roast Chicken With Honey

• Servings: 2 • Preparation time: 1h • Cook time: 15 minutes •

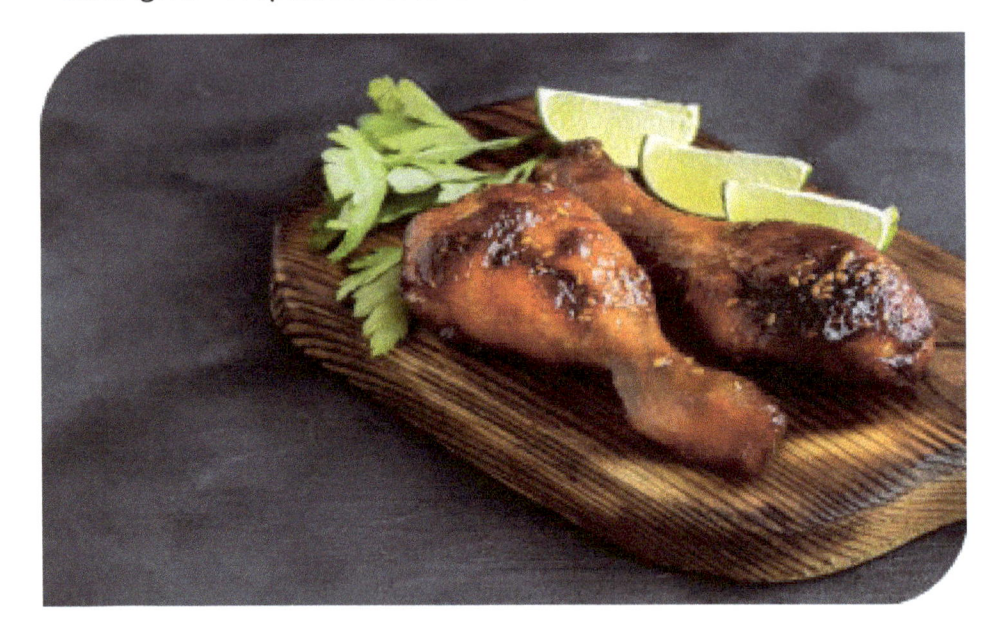

HONEYED

Ingredients

- 9 tsp of honey, and a little more sprinkle
- 3 tsp of soy sauce
- 1 lemon, in juice
- 2 garlic cloves, minced
- 4 boneless chicken thighs, skinned
- Salt to taste
- lemon wedges, to garnish

Steps to Cook

1. Put the honey, lemon juice, soy sauce, and garlic in a bowl and mix. Soak chicken and marinade for up to 1 hour.

2. Select Preheat, in the air fryer adjust the temperature to 195°C and press Start/Pause.

3. Place the chicken thighs in the preheated air fryer.

4. Select Chicken, set the time to 15 minutes and press

5. Start/Pause.

6. Remove the baskets from the air fryer when there are 5 minutes left on the timer. Cover the chicken with more marinated and returns the baskets to finish cooking. Season with salt, drizzle a little honey and garnish with lemon wedges.

Nutritional Information

- Calories: 200
- Carbohydrates: 22g
- Fat: 12g
- Protein: 3g
- Sugar: 5g
- Cholesterol: 15mg

Homemade Potatoes

• Servings: 2 • Preparation time: 5 minutes • Cook time: 25 minutes •

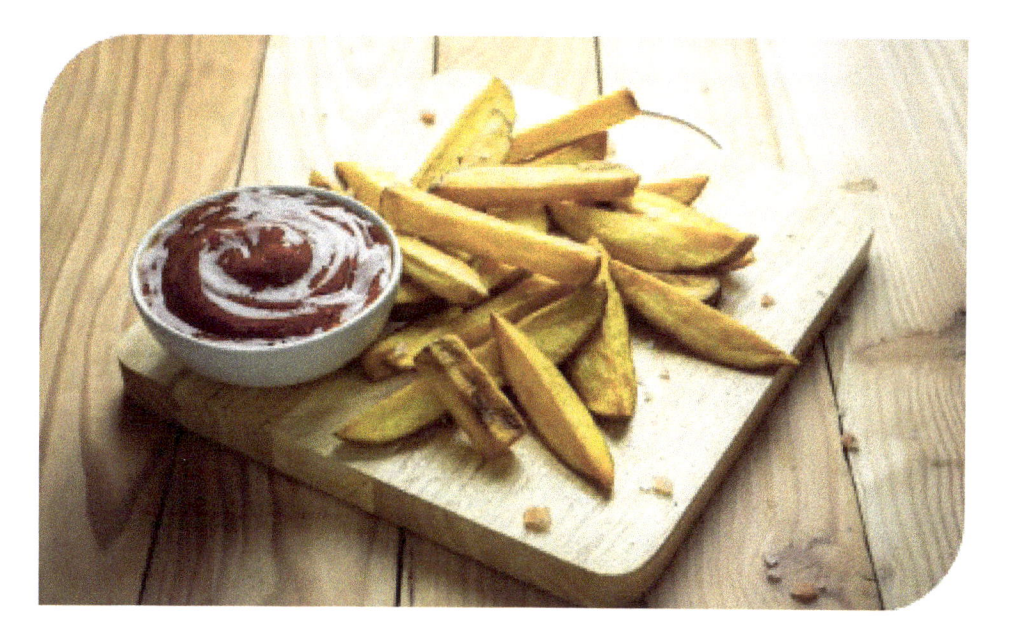

CRISPY

Ingredients

- 300 g natural potatoes
- 1 tbsp olive oil
- 1 tbsp salt
- 1 tbsp pepper

to add more flavor:

- 1 tbsp onion powder (optional)
- 1 tbsp dry parsley (optional)
- 1 tbsp Paprika (optional)
- 1 tbsp Curcuma (optional)

Steps to Cook

1. Choose some natural potatoes.

2. Peel and cut the potatoes: try to cut the potatoes to the same thickness for a complete and uniform cooking.

3. Soak the potatoes in cold water.

4. Pour the cut potatoes into a bowl: add all the ingredients, the olive oil and mix. (The tablespoon of oil helps the seasonings stick to the potatoes.)

5. Transfer the potatoes to the Air fryer container. Set the temperature to 200ºC for 16-20 minutes. (Check after 10min.

6. At the end of cooking your home fries will be ready to eat.

Nutritional Information

- Calories: 77
- Carbohydrates: 17.47g
- Fat: 0.09g
- Protein: 2.02g
- Sugar: 0.78g
- Cholesterol: 0mg

Air Fryer Cookbook

Perfect Fillet with Garlic Butter and Herbs

• Servings: 4 • Preparation time: 2 minutes • Cook time: 17 minutes •

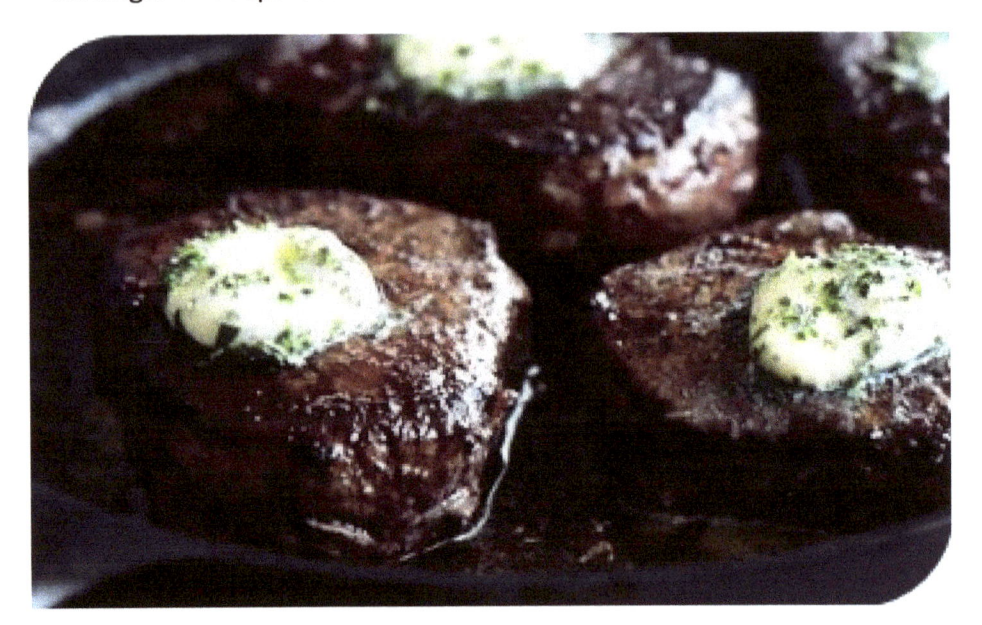

CHOCOLATY

Ingredients

- 2 8 oz Ribeye fillets
- Salt
- freshly ground black pepper
- olive oil
- Garlic butter
- 1 stick of unsalted butter, softened
- 2 tbsp chopped fresh parsley
- 2 tsp minced garlic
- 1 tsp Worcestershire sauce
- ½ teaspoon salt

Steps to Cook

1. Prepare the garlic butter by mixing butter, parsley, garlic, Worcestershire sauce and salt until well combined. Place on parchment paper and roll it on a log. Refrigerate until ready for use.

2. Remove the fillet from the fridge and let it sit at room temperature for 20 minutes. Rub a little olive oil on both sides of the steak and season with salt and freshly ground black pepper. Grease the fryer basket by rubbing a little oil into the basket. Preheat the air fryer to 400ºF. Once preheated, place the fillets in the fryer and cook for 12 minutes, turning them in half. Remove from fryer and let sit for 5 minutes. Top with garlic butter.

Nutritional Information

- Calories: 667
- Carbohydrates: 1g
- Fat: 53g
- Protein: 45g
- Sugar: 0g
- Cholesterol: 300mg

Cordon Bleu Style Stuffed Chicken Breast

• Servings: 1 • Preparation time: 15 minutes • Cook time: 20 minutes •

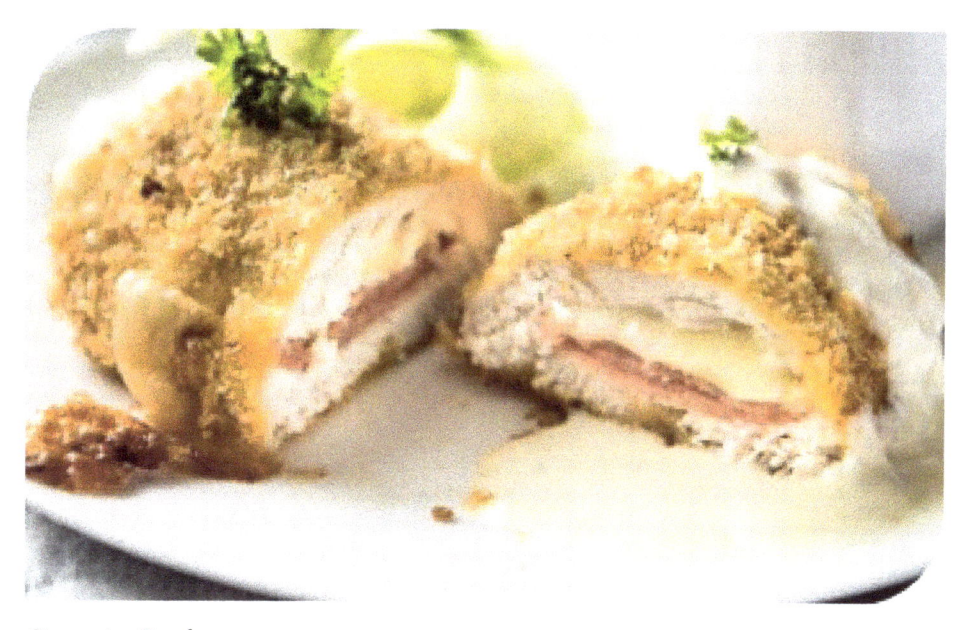

JUICY
───

Ingredients

- ½ lb Chicken breast.
- ½ lb Ham slices
- 5 slices melted cheese, gruyere or mozzarella
- 2 eggs
- Ground bread
- Salt to taste

Steps to Cook

1. Cut the chicken breasts as thin as possible.

2. Wrap the cheese inside the ham slices.

3. Put the chicken sheets between two plastic sheets.

4. And crush the chicken with a mallet to make it thinner. Put the cheese wrapped in ham on the chicken breast slices and wrap.

5. Stir the two eggs and they are very well beaten.

6. Make a bowl of breadcrumbs or breadcrumbs.

7. Pass the chicken breasts over the breadcrumbs first.

8. Then soak them in the beaten egg.

9. And run them over the breading again.

10. Finally, spray the chicken breasts with oil and put them in the Air fryer at 200ºC for 20 minutes.

Nutritional Information

- Calories: 330
- Carbohydrates: 18g
- Fat: 14g
- Protein: 32g
- Sugar: 2g
- Cholesterol: 85mg

Air Fryer Cookbook

Tikka Chicken

• Servings: 2 • Preparation time: 1h • Cook time: 20 minutes •

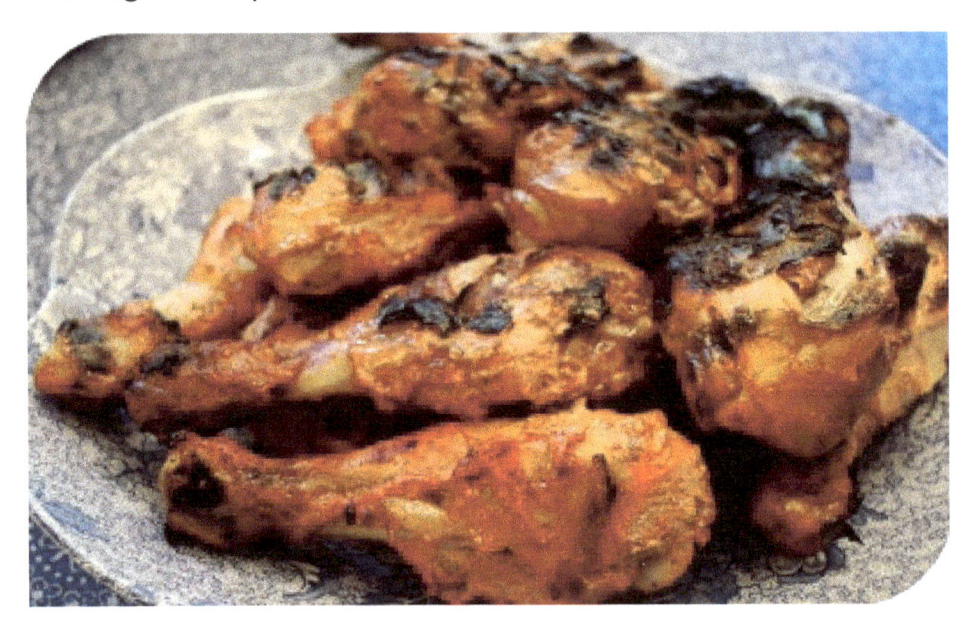

TOASTED

Ingredients

- 1/3 cup coconut milk
- 1/8 oz. tomato paste
- ½ tsp of garam marsala
- 1/3 tsp cumin
- ½ tsp turmeric
- 1/3 tsp cardamom
- ½ tsp garlic powder
- 1 oz. ginger, grated
- 1 tsp of salt
- 4 chicken thighs

Steps to Cook

1. Put everything except chicken in a bowl and mix.

2. Soak the chicken feet in the coconut marinade and mix until the legs are well covered. Marinate for up to 1 hour.

3. Select Preheat, in the air fryer adjust the temperature to 175°C and press Start/Pause.

4. Remove the chicken legs from the refrigerator and place them in the preheated air fryer.

5. Cook at 175°C for 20 minutes.

6. Serve with what you want even with steamed basmati rice.

Nutritional Information

- Calories: 290
- Carbohydrates: 11g
- Fat: 12g
- Protein: 19g
- Sugar: 5g
- Cholesterol: 218mg

Spinach Stuffed Chicken

• Servings: 3-4 • Preparation time: 10 minutes • Cook time: 15 minutes •

Steps to Cook

1. Heat the olive oil in a medium flame skillet

2. Add the spinach to the pan with some salt and pepper. Stir constantly until spinach is cooked and drained. (2 to 3 minutes)

3. Transfer the spinach to a medium bowl to stir with the cream cheese, mozzarella and tablespoon of garlic powder.

Chicken Instructions:

4. Cut chicken breast in half

5. Make a cut in the middle of the breast to form a hole where we are going to put the spinach.

6. Place the spinach in the center of the breast

Breaded:

7. In three different bowls you will place:

8. 1 bowl: flour

9. 2 bowl: beaten eggs

10. 3 bowl: Ground bread

11. Then, in that order we are going to smear the chicken breast in the flour, then in the beaten eggs and finally in the breadcrumbs.

Use the air fryer:

12. You can spray a little oil on the basket of your air fryer to prevent food from sticking.

13. Put the spinach stuffed chicken into your air fryer at a temperature of 150ºC for 10 minutes

14. At the end of the 10 minutes turn the chicken breast and cook for 5 more minutes at the same temperature.

YUMMY

Ingredients

- 1 tbsp olive oil
- 5 oz baby spinach
- 8 oz cream cheese
- 1 cup grated mozzarella cheese
- 1 tbsp garlic powder
- 7 pieces boneless skinless chicken breast
- 1 cup all-purpose flour
- 3 pieces eggs
- 2 cups breadcrumbs/breadcrumbs

Nutritional Information

- Calories: 293.9
- Carbohydrates: 6.5g
- Fat: 18g
- Protein: 26.3g
- Sugar: 1.4g
- Cholesterol: 67.1mg

Air Fryer Cookbook

Breaded Fish

• Servings: 1 • Preparation time: 30 minutes • Cook time: 16 minutes •

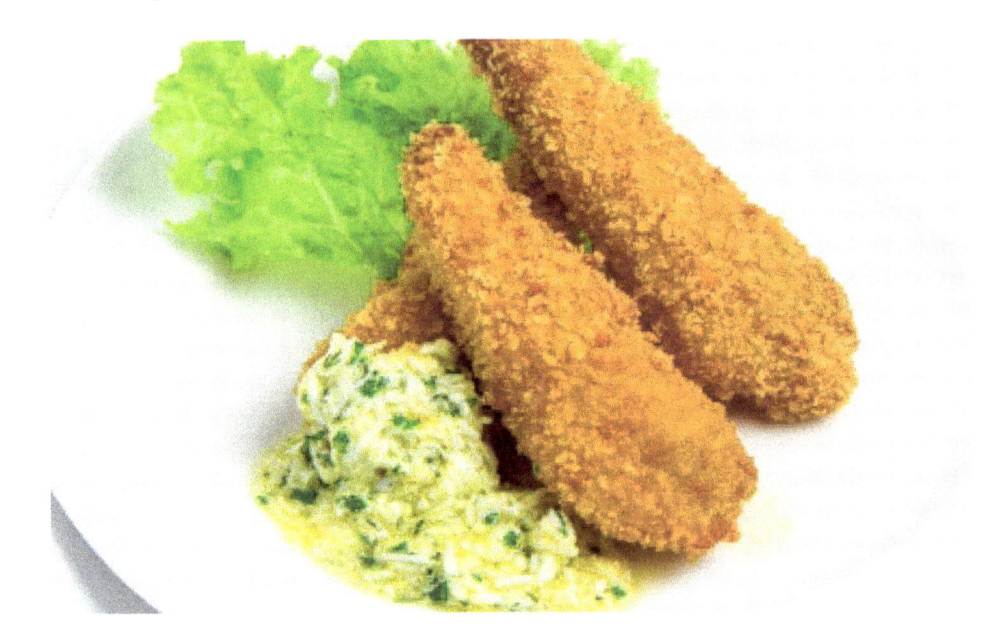

TOASTED

Ingredients

- 3 pieces of fish
- ½ tbsp or salt to taste
- 1 tbsp pepper
- 1 tbsp ground garlic
- 1 ½ tbsp olive oil

You can prepare it with:

- ½ Cup Ground bread
- or
- ½ Cup Wheat flour

Steps to Cook

1. Prepare your fish with the garlic, salt and pepper.
2. In a pot or bowl prepare the flour with the eggs.
3. Pass the fish through the breaded and check that it adheres well.
4. And put the pieces in the air fryer
5. Set the temperature of your air fryer to 350ºF.
6. Turn your fryer on in 8 minutes.
7. Turn the Fish over, check how much it is missing and put it around 8 minutes again.

Nutritional Information

- Calories: 260
- Carbohydrates: 23g
- Fat: 12g
- Protein: 16g
- Sugar: 1g
- Cholesterol: 45mg

Japanese-Style Meatballs

• Servings: 4 • Preparation time: 15 minutes • Cook time: 10 minutes •

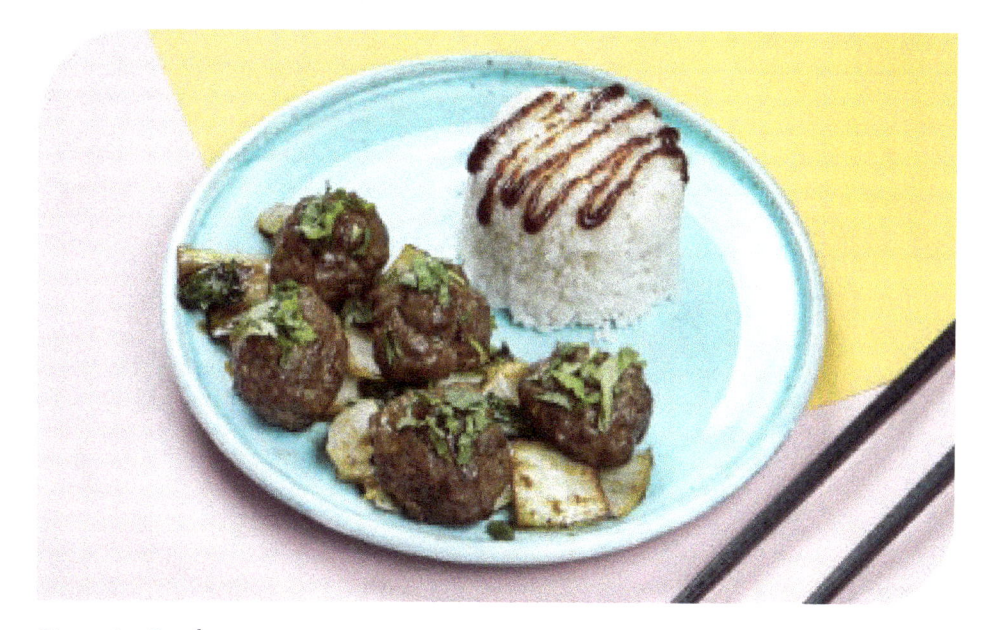

Ingredients

- 16 oz ground beef
- 3 tsp sesame oil 18 g miso paste
- 10 fresh mint leaves, finely chopped
- 4 chives, finely chopped
- 1 tsp of salt
- ¼ tsp of black pepper
- 9 tsp of soy sauce
- 9 tsp of mirin
- 9 tsp of water
- 1 tsp of brown sugar

Steps to Cook

1. Mix the ground beef, sesame oil, miso paste, mint leaves, chives, salt and pepper until everything is well combined. Add a small amount of sesame oil to your hands and create 51mm dumplings with the mixture. You should be left with 8 meatballs approximately.

2. Let the meatballs cool in the refrigerator for 10 minutes. Create the sauce by mixing the soy sauce, mirin, water and brown sugar. Leave aside.

3. Select Preheat on the air fryer and press

4. Start/Pause. Arrange the chilled meatballs in the preheated air fryer.

5. Select Fillet, set the time to 10 minutes and press Start/Pause. Liberally brush the meatballs with the glaze every 2 minutes.

Nutritional Information

- Calories: 420
- Carbohydrates: 61g
- Fat: 11g
- Protein: 20g
- Sugar: 16g
- Cholesterol: 45mg

Air Fryer Cookbook

Picanha Steak Cut

• Servings: 4 • Preparation time: 15 minutes • Cook time: 15 minutes •

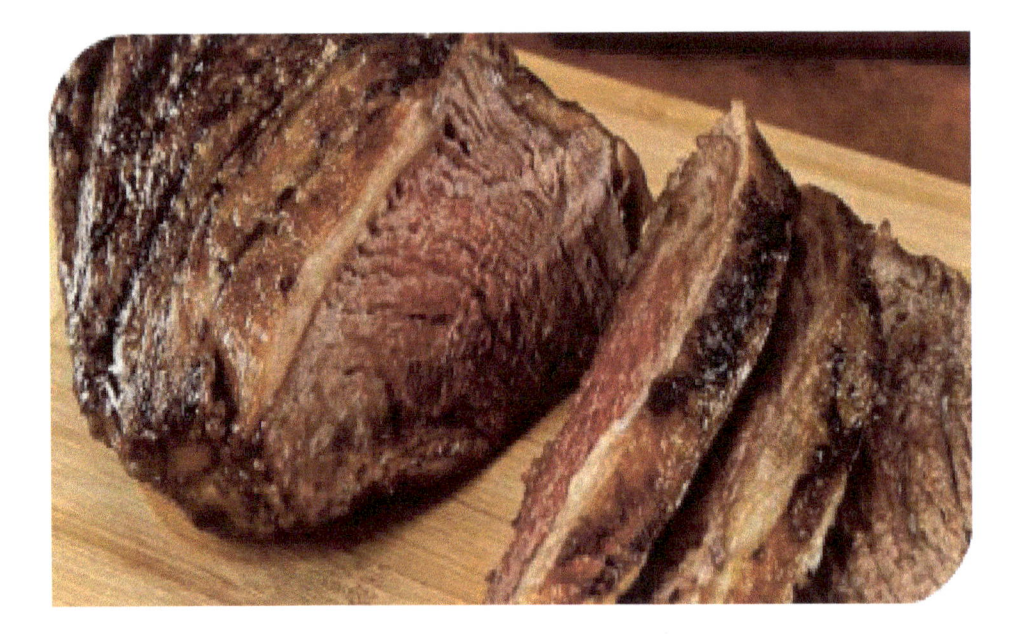

AMAZINGLY DELICIOUS

Ingredients

- 1 pound beef (1 piece)
- Salt: It can be ground or in pieces.
- Ground pepper

Steps to Cook

1. Cut with a knife, on top of the fat, making straight lines to form a kind of diamond. (Lines inclined to the left and lines inclined to the right).

2. Season with salt and pepper all the picanha.

3. Put it in your air fryer with the facing up.

4. Cooking at 150°C for 10 minutes with the fat on top. At the end turn the cut of picanha and add 5 more minutes.

5. At the end, let picanha rest for 2 to 4 minutes so that it does not drain when cut.

....

Nutritional Information

- Calories: 390
- Carbohydrates: 1.3g
- Fat: 24g
- Protein: 42g
- Sugar: 0g
- Cholesterol: 135mg

Brussels Sprouts

• Servings: 2 • Preparation time: 5 minutes • Cook time: 8 minutes •

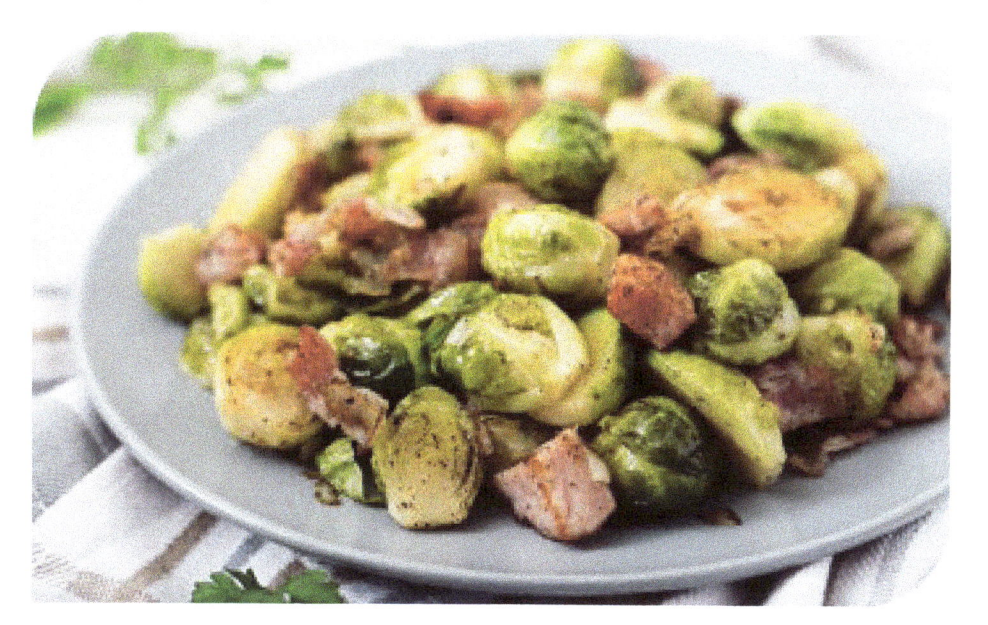

TASTY

Ingredients

- ½ oz. brussels sprouts, halved
- 2 strips of bacon, diced
- 4 tsp olive oil
- ½ tsp garlic powder
- Salt and pepper to taste
- 1 tsp Parmesan cheese, freshly grated

Steps to Cook

1. Select Preheat on the air fryer and press Start/Pause.

2. Cut the stems of the Brussels sprouts and then cut them in half.

3. Combine the halves of the cabbage sprouts, olive oil, garlic powder, salt, and pepper in a bowl.

4. Add the mixture to the preheated air fryer.

5. Select Tubers and press Start/Pause. Make sure to shake the baskets halfway through cooking.

6. Grate Parmesan cheese for garnish and serve.

Nutritional Information

- Calories: 60
- Carbohydrates: 12g
- Fat: 3g
- Protein: 4.3g
- Sugar: 2.9g
- Cholesterol: 0mg

Air Fryer Cookbook

Guava And Cheese Dumplings

• Servings: 4 • Preparation time: 5 minutes • Cook time: 23 minutes •

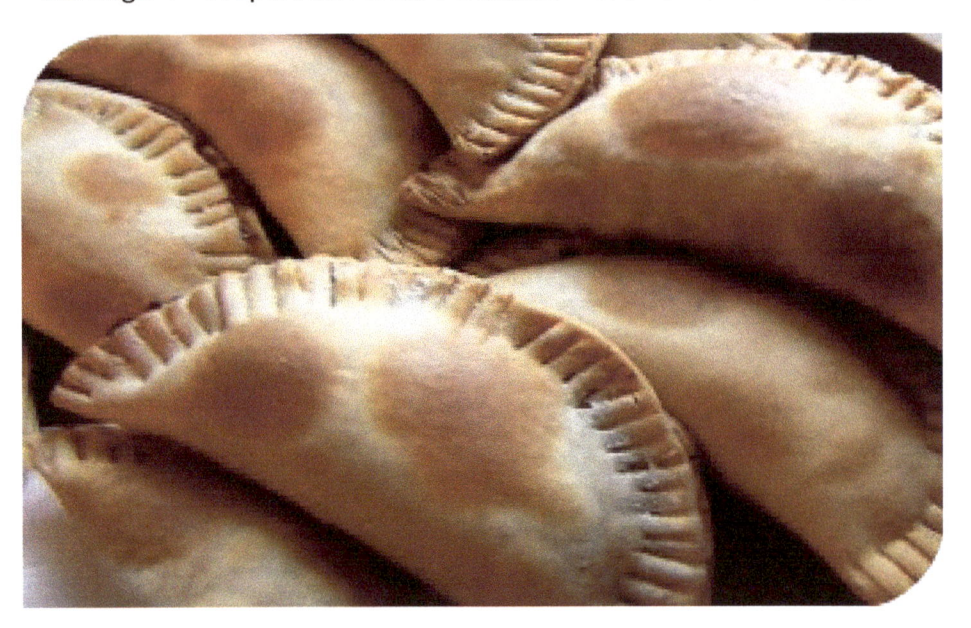

FRUITY

Ingredients

• Templates for cupcakes and dumplings

• cheese of your choice (can be American or white)

• guava paste

Steps to Cook

1. Preheat the air fryer to 325ºF for 8 minutes. Spray the basket with cooking oil

2. Cut the cheese and the guava paste into cubes.

3. Take a piece of cheese and place it in the middle of the tortilla on the dumplings template. On top of this, put some cubes of the guava paste. Fold half of the dough over the ingredients and press the corners with a fork to seal them. Repeat with the other ingredients.

Nutritional Information

- Calories: 115
- Carbohydrates: 14g
- Fat: 5g
- Protein: 4g
- Sugar: 0g
- Cholesterol: 295mg

Garlic Bread

• Servings: 2 • Preparation time: 1h • Cook time: 15 minutes •

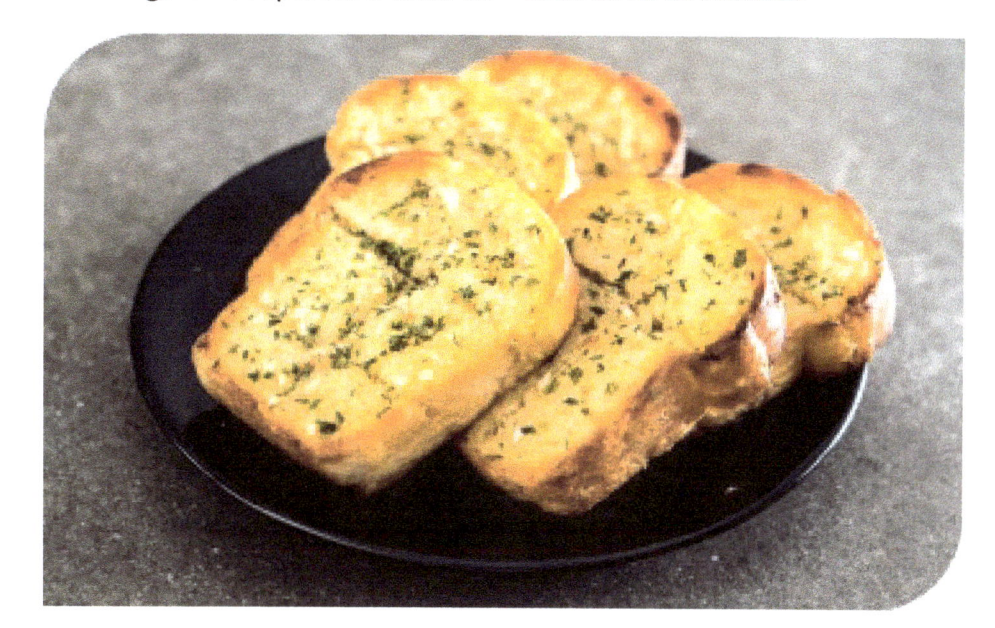

CRUNCHY

Ingredients

- 1 French baguette (305 mm), cut lengthwise and widthwise
- 4 garlic cloves, minced
- 1 ½ oz. butter, room temperature
- 3 tsp olive oil
- 2 tsp Parmesan cheese, grated
- 1 ½ tsp parsley, freshly chopped

Steps to Cook

1. Cut the baguette in half lengthwise, then divide each piece in half widthwise, creating 4 slices 152mm long.

2 Select Preheat on the air fryer, set it to 160 ° C and press Start/Pause.

3. Combine garlic, butter, and olive oil to form a paste.

4. Spread the pasta evenly on the bread and sprinkle with Parmesan cheese.

5. Place the bread in the preheated air fryer.

6. Select Pan and press Start/Pause.

7. Garnish with freshly chopped parsley when you're done cooking.

Nutritional Information

- Calories: 350
- Carbohydrates: 42g
- Fat: 17g
- Protein: 8.4g
- Sugar: 3.7g
- Cholesterol: 45mg

Potato Fillings

• Servings: 4 • Preparation time: 10 minutes • Cook time: 12 minutes •

Ingredients

- 4 potatoes
- 1 ½ cup of medium prepared ground beef
- 2 eggs
- 1 cup of ground cookie
- 1 cup baking flour
- Oil of your choice
- salt and pepper
- ½ cup grated Parmesan cheese
- parsley for decoration

Steps to Cook

1. Peel and cut the potatoes into equal pieces - preferably small - to ensure each cooks equally and boils until smooth. Once they are ready, remove them from the water, drain and transfer them to a medium bowl. Once in the container, with a fork, mash them until smooth. Add salt and pepper to taste.

2. In a separate bowl, beat the two eggs and set aside. Prepare the flour and the cracked cookie on separate plates.

3. Put a little flour in the palm of your hand, to create a protective layer, and so the potato mixture does not stick. With a spoon, take a reasonable amount and crush it in your hand. Then, fill with a little ground beef, just enough so that the potato won't open, add more potato mixture on top of the meat and turn it into a ball.

4. Pass the filling first through the flour and then through the egg. Finally, you can transfer it to the plate with the ground biscuits and Parmesan cheese. Repeat the same process with the following.

5. Once you have the potato fillings ready, with a kitchen brush, rub a little oil of your choice on top, to achieve a crispy consistency. Cook in the air fryer at a temperature of 400ºF for 12 minutes.

Nutritional Information

- Calories: 220
- Carbohydrates: 30.6g
- Fat: 15.9g
- Protein: 8.1g
- Sugar: 10g
- Cholesterol: 63mg

Roasted Aubergine

• Servings: 2 • Preparation time: 5 minutes• Cook time: 10 minutes •

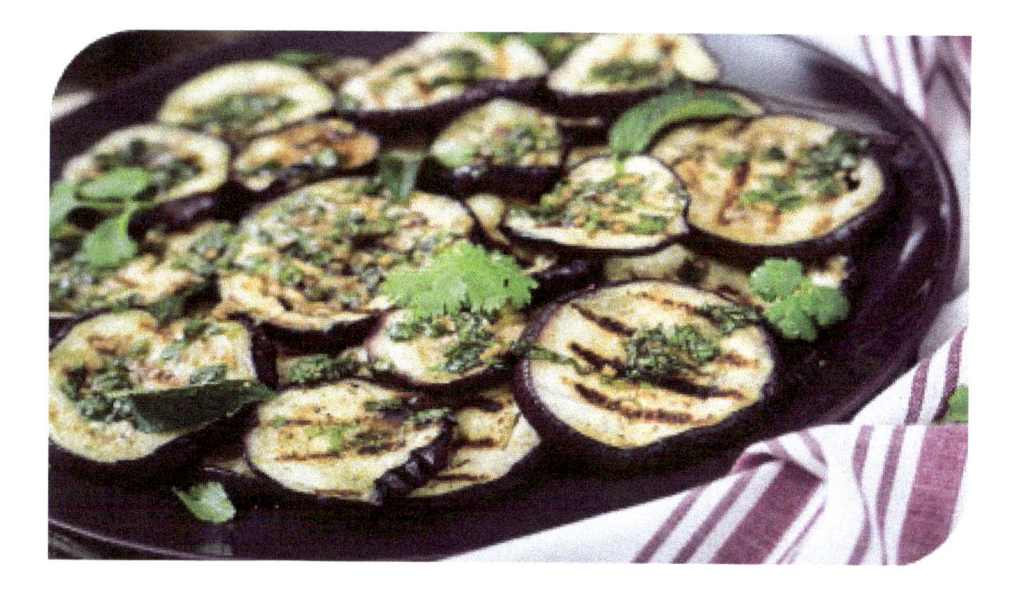

SALTY

Ingredients

- 1 Japanese aubergine, cut into 13 mm thick slices
- 6 tsp olive oil
- ½ tsp of salt
- 1/3 tsp garlic powder
- ¼ tsp black pepper
- ¼ tsp onion powder
- ¼ tsp of ground cumin

Steps to Cook

1. Select Preheat on the air fryer and press Start/Pause.

2. Cut the peeled eggplant into 13mm thick slices.

3. Combine oil and seasonings in large bowl until well combined, and mix eggplant until all pieces are well covered.

4. Place the eggplant in the preheated air fryer and cook at 205°C for 10 minutes.

Nutritional Information

- Calories: 49.6
- Carbohydrates: 9.4g
- Fat: 1.4g
- Protein: 1.6g
- Sugar: 0g
- Cholesterol: 0mg

Fried Cutlets

• Servings: 4 • Preparation time: 10 minutes • Cook time: 5 minutes •

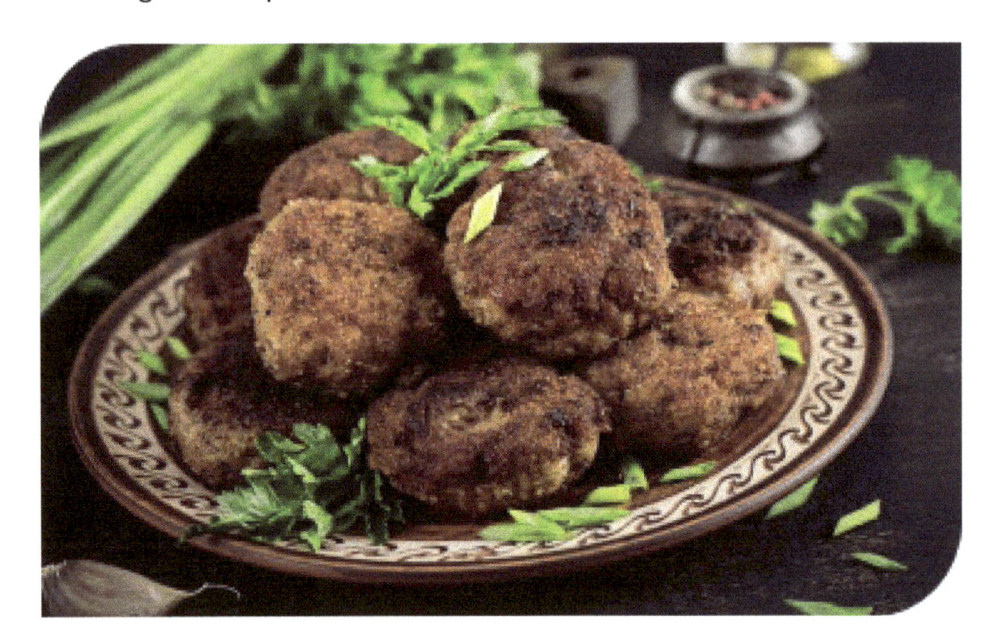

APPETIZING

Ingredients

- 3 cloves minced garlic
- 2 tbsp of olive oil
- 1 tbsp of marinade
- 4 thawed pork chops

Steps to Cook

1. Firstly, gather the ingredients.

2. Mix the ground garlic cloves, the marinade and the oil. Then apply this mixture on the chops.

3. Select the frying mode of your air fryer.

4. Select 360°C for 35 minutes.

Nutritional Information

- Calories: 271
- Carbohydrates: 16g
- Fat: 8.4g
- Protein: 31g
- Sugar: 0.9g
- Cholesterol: 148mg

Grilled Pumpkin

• Servings: 2 • Preparation time: 10minutes • Cook time: 12 minutes •

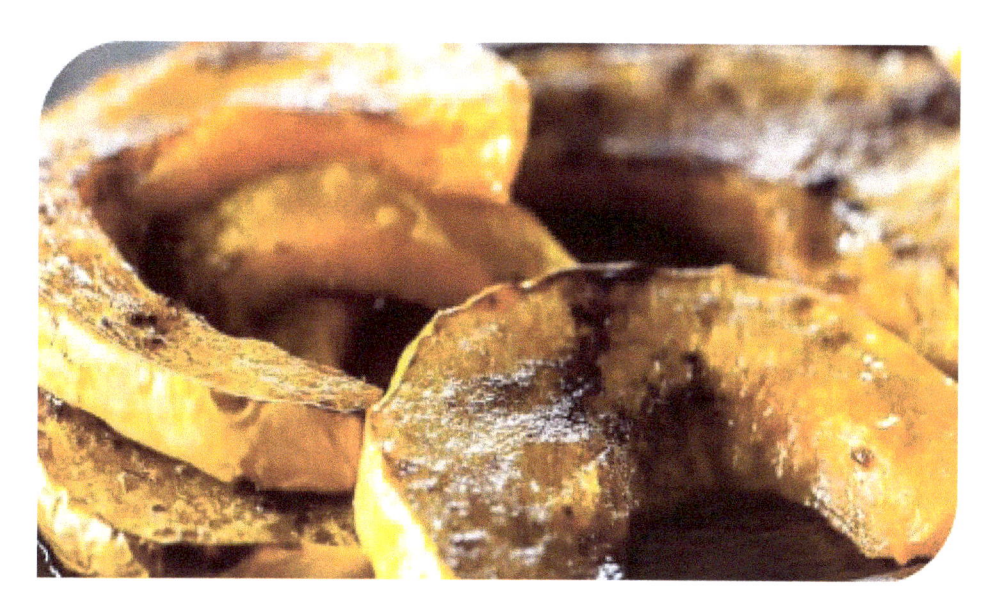

HOT

Ingredients

- 1 pumpkin, peeled, seeded and cut into 25mm cubes
- 3 tsp of olive oil, plus a little more to spray
- ¼ tsp thyme leaves
- 1 tsp of salt
- ¼ tsp black pepper

Steps to Cook

1. Select Preheat on the air fryer and press Start/Pause.

2. Cover the pumpkin cubes seasoned with olive oil and season with thyme, salt and pepper.

3. Add the seasoned squash to the preheated air fryer.

4. Select 200ºC for 12 minutes. Make sure to shake the baskets halfway through cooking.

5. Drizzle with olive oil when it is done and serve.

Nutritional Information

- Calories: 28
- Carbohydrates: 4g
- Fat: 0g
- Protein: 1g
- Sugar: 2g
- Cholesterol: 300mg

Chicken Greaves

• Servings: 4 • Preparation time: 1-2h • Cook time: 25 minutes •

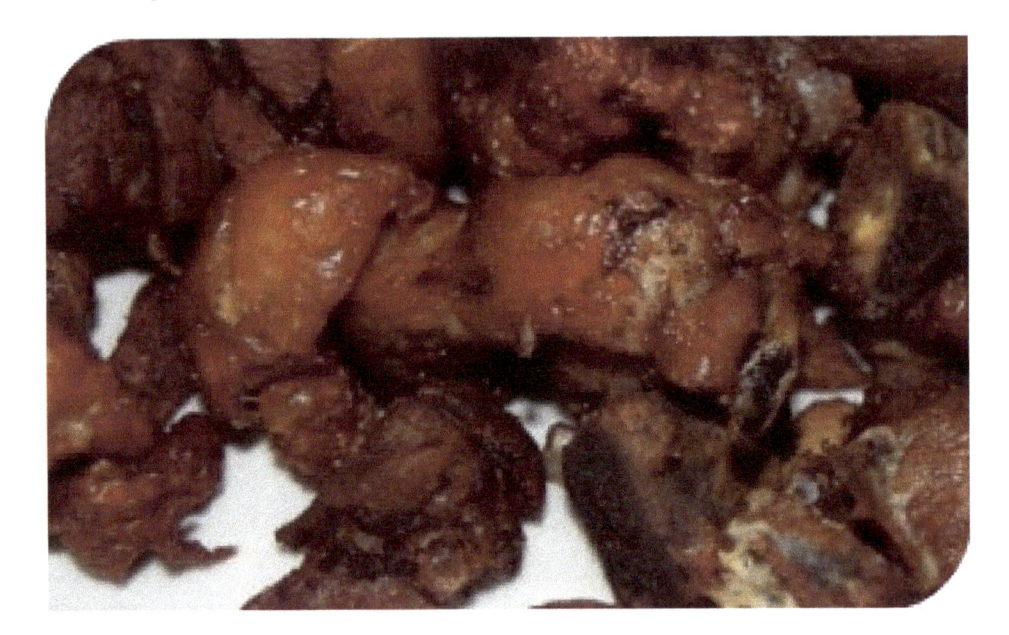

EXTRAORDINARY

Ingredients

- ½ unit of chicken
- ¼ of Cup of olive oil
- 1 tsp of vinegar
- 1 envelope of seasoning
- 1 tsp minced garlic
- lemon to taste

Steps to Cook

1. Wash and chop the chicken into pieces. Then sprinkle some marinade on it.

2. In a container mix the rest of the ingredients. Once ready, pour the liquid over the chicken.

3. Let marinate in the refrigerator for 2 to 5 hours.

To cook:

4. Place in the air fryer at 390°F for 13 minutes.

5. When the time is up, move the chicken pieces and cook for 12 more minutes.

Nutritional Information

- Calories: 190
- Carbohydrates: 0g
- Fat: 11g
- Protein: 20g
- Sugar: 0g
- Cholesterol: 65mg

Grilled Cauliflower

• Servings: 4 • Preparation time: 2 minutes • Cook time: 10 minutes •

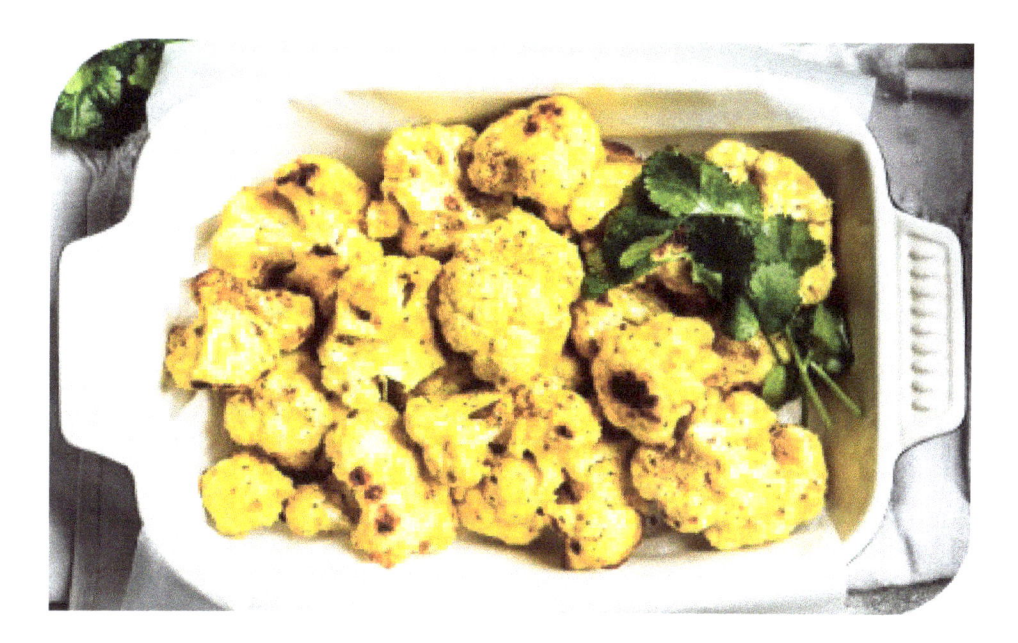

TOASTED

Ingredients

- ½ lb cauliflower
- 2 tsp olive oil
- ½ tsp of salt
- ¼ tsp black pepper

Steps to Cook

1. Select Preheat on the air fryer, set it to 150°C, and press Start/Pause.

2. Place the cauliflower florets in a container, drizzle with olive oil and season with salt and pepper, evenly covering the florets.

3. Add the cauliflower to the preheated air fryer.

4. Select 150ºC for 10 minutes.

Nutritional Information

- Calories: 271
- Carbohydrates: 9g
- Fat: 25.2g
- Protein: 5.8g
- Sugar: 3.9g
- Cholesterol: 66.4mg

Air Fryer Cookbook

Pork Taquitos

• Servings: 2-4 • Preparation time: 5 minutes • Cook time: 10 minutes •

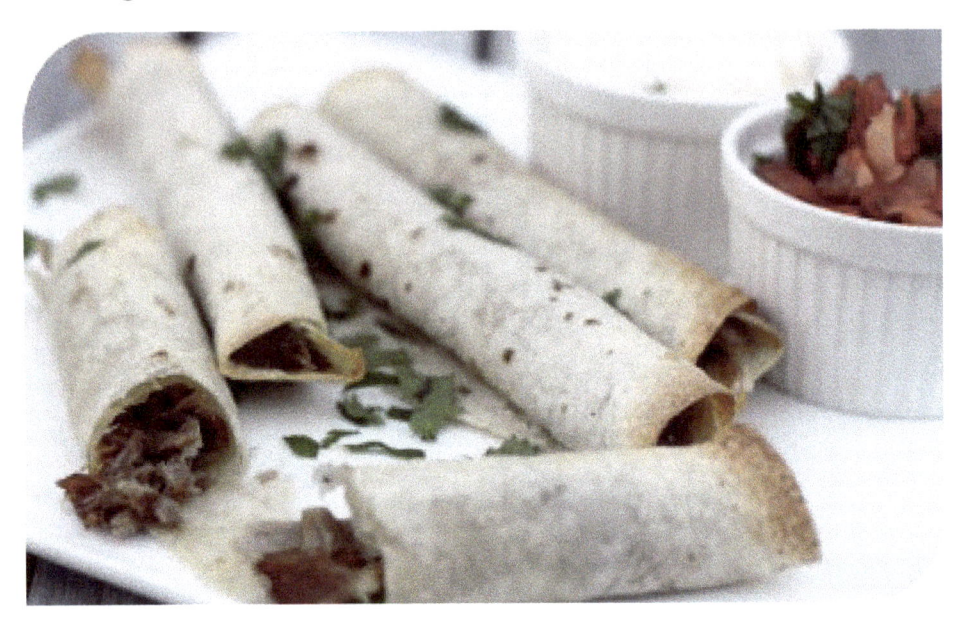

AMAZINGLY DELICIOUS

Ingredients

- 3 cups minced pork loin (previously cooked)
- juice of a lemon
- 10 templates
- 2 cups of mozzarella cheese
- cooking spray
- sauce to taste
- sour cream to taste

Steps to Cook

1. Preheat fryer to 380ºF. Meanwhile, microwave insoles for 10 seconds.

2. On the other hand, in a container add the pork with a pinch of lemon.

3. Then add the pulled pork and cheese to the template. Roll up the template and close.

4. Once ready, add spray over these and put in the air fryer for 10 minutes (remember to brown each side!).

Nutritional Information

- Calories: 210
- Carbohydrates: 25g
- Fat: 9g
- Protein: 7g
- Sugar: 2g
- Cholesterol: 10mg

Grilled Broccoli

• Servings: 3 • Preparation time: 3 minutes • Cook time: 10 minutes •

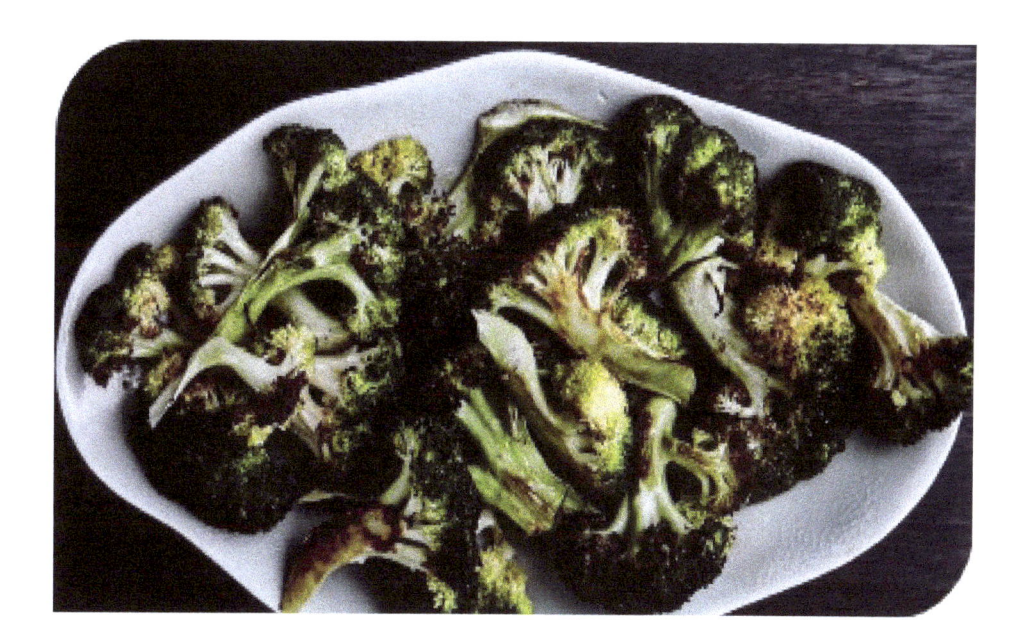

Ingredients

- 1 large head broccoli, cut into florets
- 3 tsp olive oil
- ½ tsp garlic powder
- ½ tsp of salt
- ¼ tsp black pepper

Steps to Cook

1. Select Preheat on the air fryer, set it to 150°C, and press Start/Pause.
2. Drizzle the broccoli pieces with olive oil and mix until well covered.
3. Mix the broccoli with the seasonings.
4. Add the broccoli to the preheated air fryer.
5. Cook at the same temperature for 10 minutes

Nutritional Information

- Calories: 80
- Carbohydrates: 11g
- Fat: 3g
- Protein: 3g
- Sugar: 1g
- Cholesterol: 0mg

Classic Bacon

• Servings: 2 • Preparation time: 3 minutes • Cook time: 10-15 minutes •

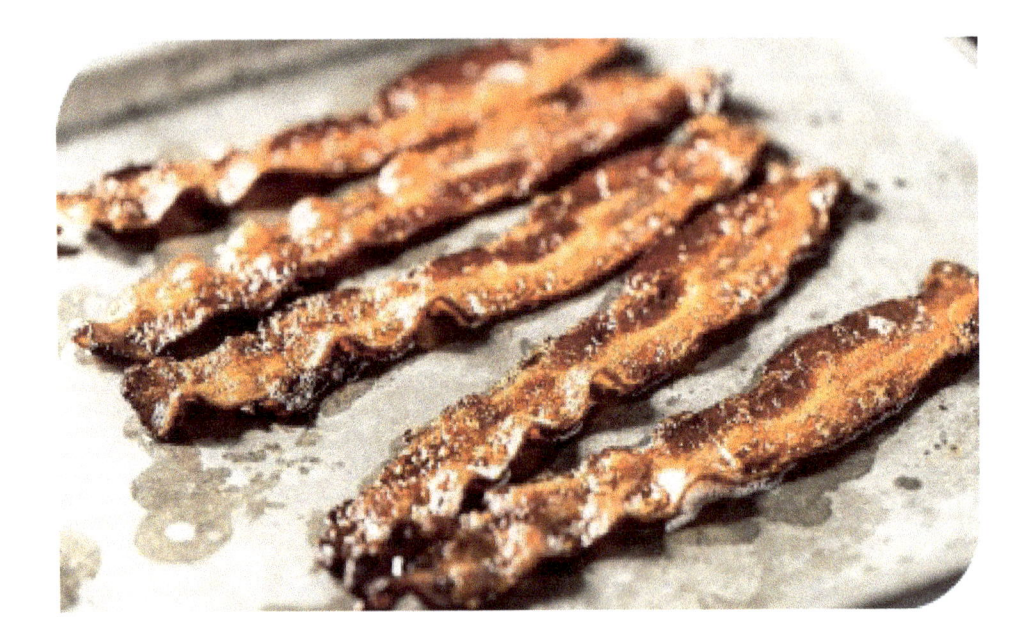

TASTEFUL

Ingredients

- 7 to 8 bacon flakes

Steps to Cook

1. In the basket of your fryer, place the chips vertically and a few horizontally.

2. Then, set the temperature to 350ºF.

3. Cook for 10 to 15 minutes.

4. Stop time and see how golden your bacon has been.

5. If you want it to be crispier, flip the food over and cook once more.

Nutritional Information

- Calories: 161
- Carbohydrates: 0.6g
- Fat: 12g
- Protein: 12g
- Sugar: 0g
- Cholesterol: 34mg

Grilled Carrots with Honey

• Servings: 2-4 • Preparation time: 5 minutes • Cook time: 12 minutes •

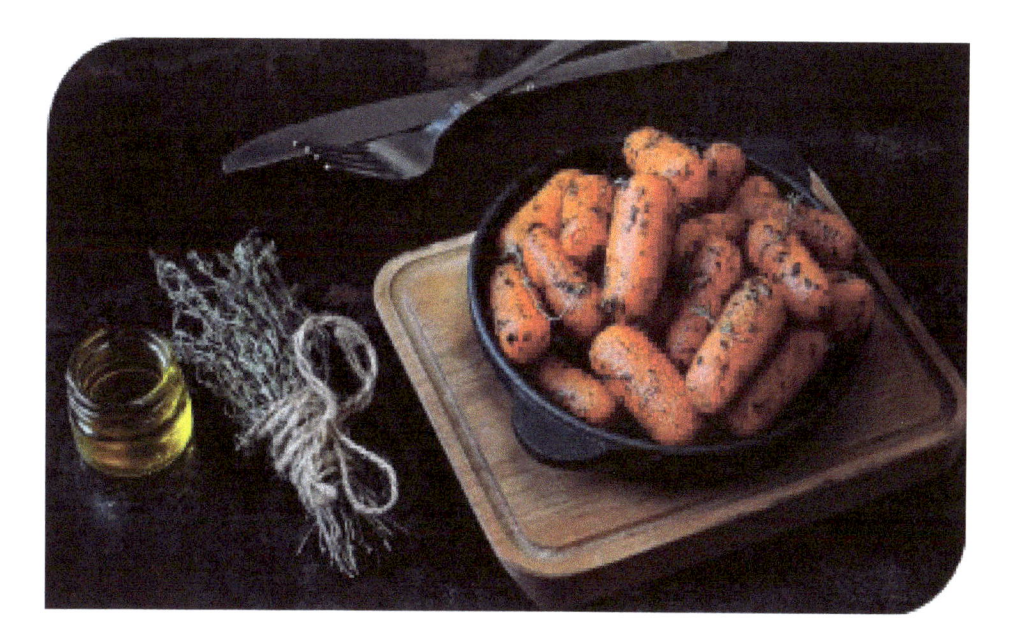

HONEYED

Ingredients

- 1 lb rainbow carrots, peeled and washed
- 3 tsp olive oil
- 6 tsp of honey
- 2 sprigs of fresh thyme
- Salt and pepper to taste

Steps to Cook

1. Wash the carrots and pat dry with a paper towel. Leave aside.
2. Select Preheat on the air fryer and press Start/Pause.
3. Place the carrots in a bowl with olive oil, honey, thyme, salt, and pepper.
4. Select 150ºC for 12 minutes. Make sure to shake the baskets halfway through cooking.
5. Serve hot.

Nutritional Information

- Calories: 70
- Carbohydrates: 18g
- Fat: 0g
- Protein: 1g
- Sugar: 10g
- Cholesterol: 0mg

Air Fryer Cookbook

Wings in Honey and Sriracha

• Servings: 2 • Preparation time: 5 minutes • Cook time: 35 minutes •

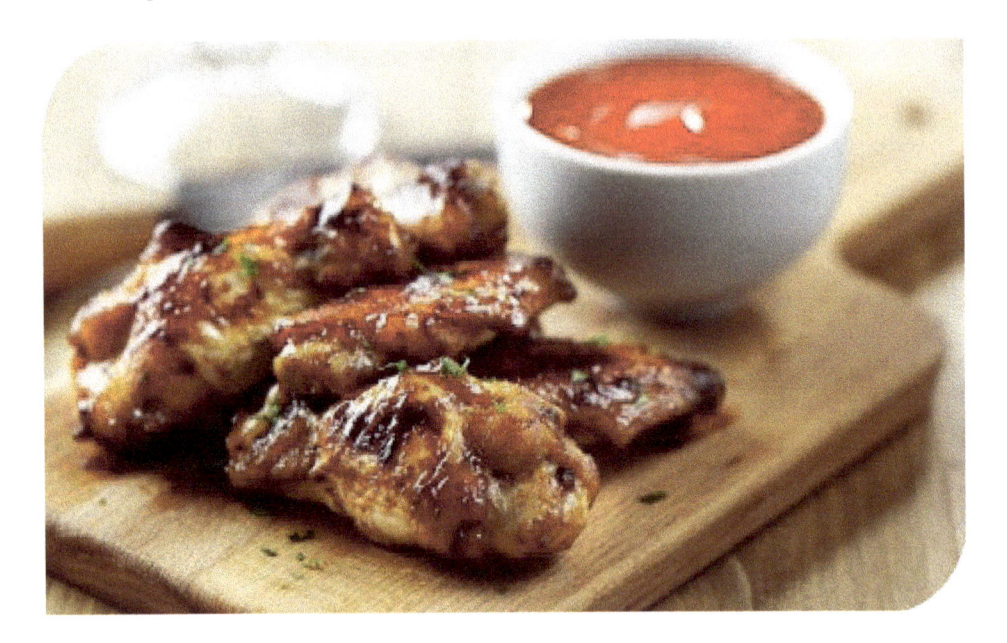

TOOTHSOME

Ingredients

- 1 lb chicken wings
- ¼ cup honey
- 2 tbsp of Sriracha sauce
- 1 ½ tbsp soy sauce
- 1 tbsp butter
- juice of ½ lemon
- coriander

Steps to Cook

1. Preheat air fryer to 360ºF.

2. Add the wings and cook for 30 minutes.

3. On the other hand, in a saucepan add honey, Sriracha and soy. Mix and cook for 3 to 5 minutes.

4. Place the wings in a deep container and then pour the sauce. Combine everything and add a little coriander.

Nutritional Information

- Calories: 190
- Carbohydrates: 18g
- Fat: 9g
- Protein: 10g
- Sugar: 4g
- Cholesterol: 275mg

Salmon with Potato

• Servings: 1-2 • Preparation time: 5minutes • Cook time: 20 minutes •

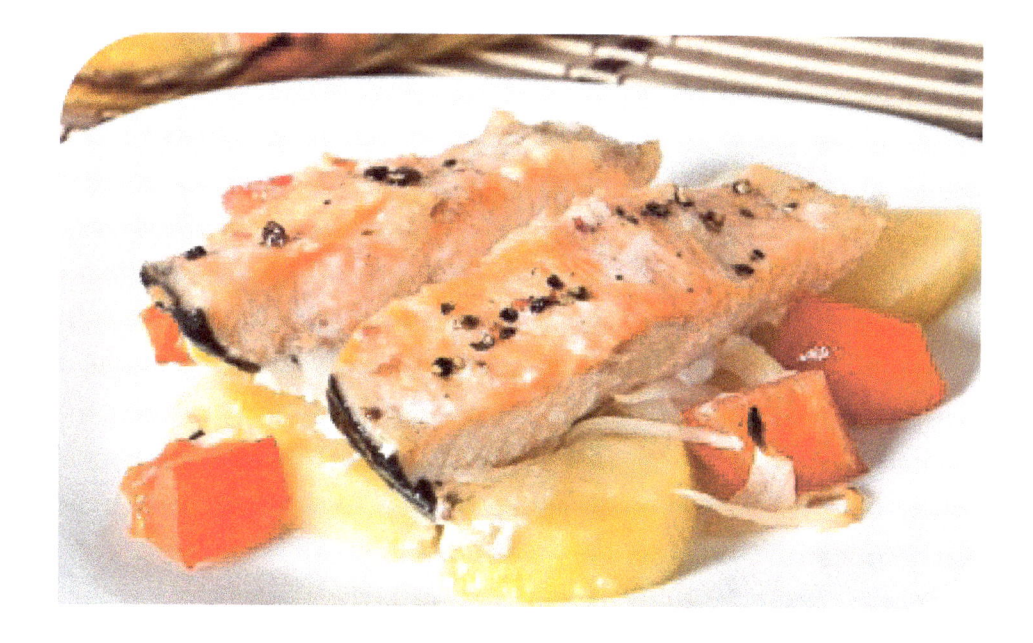

FLAVORFUL

Ingredients

- 2 salmon fillet
- Carrot
- Tomato
- Avocado
- Normal and red onion
- Vinaigrette
- Spices
- Dad

Steps to Cook

1. Prepare and marinate the fish. Heat to 200ºC, for 20 minutes in the fryer
2. Brown potatoes in deep fryer at 200ºC and stir.
3. Chop and stir the salad ingredients.

Nutritional Information

- Calories: 337.9
- Carbohydrates: 15.7g
- Fat: 16.5g
- Protein: 31.6g
- Sugar: 3.3g
- Cholesterol: 80.5mg

Air Fryer Cookbook

Roasted Potatoes

• Servings: 4 • Preparation time: 5 minutes • Cook time: 20 minutes •

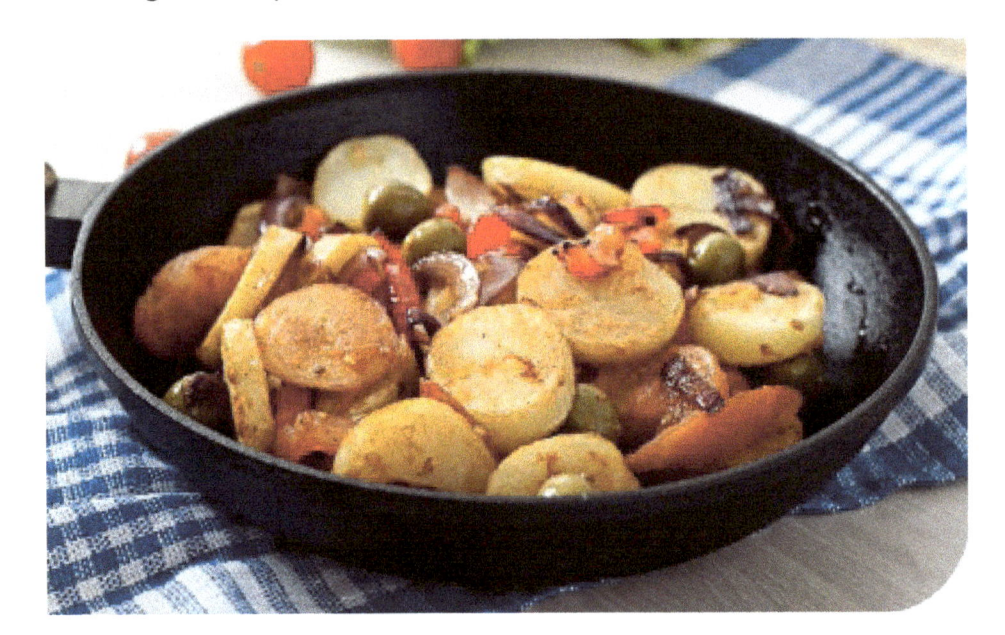

QUICK & EASY

Ingredients

- 8 oz. small fresh potatoes, cleaned and halved
- 6 tsp olive oil
- ½ tsp of salt
- ¼ tsp black pepper
- 1/3 tsp garlic powder
- ¼ tsp dried thyme
- ¼ tsp dried rosemary

Steps to Cook

1. Select Preheat on the air fryer, set it to 195°C and press Start/Pause.

2. Cover the potatoes in half with olive oil and mix the seasonings.

3. Place the potatoes in the preheated air fryer.

4. Select French Fries, set the time to 20 minutes, and press Start/Pause. Make sure to shake the baskets halfway through cooking.

Nutritional Information

- Calories: 180
- Carbohydrates: 23g
- Fat: 8.6g
- Protein: 2.7g
- Sugar: 1.7g
- Cholesterol: 0mg

Turkey Breast

• Servings: 8 • Preparation time: 5 minutes • Cook time: 55 minutes •

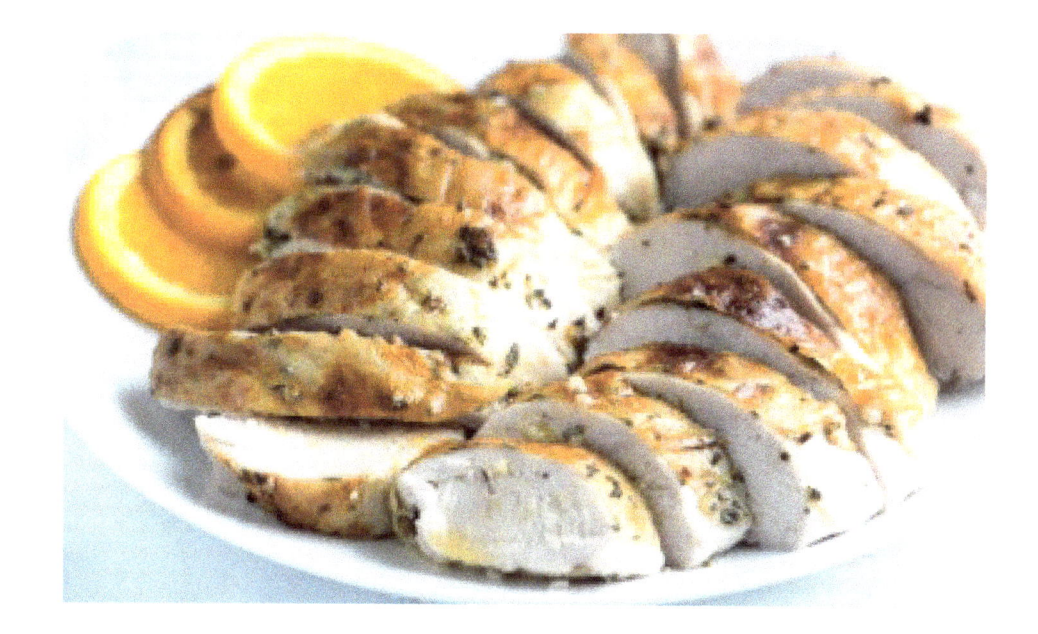

DELICIOUS

Ingredients

- 4 lbs turkey breast, bone in skin
- 1 tbsp of olive oil
- 2 tsp of kosher
- ½ tbsp dry turkey or chicken seasoning

Steps to Cook

1. Rub ½ tablespoon of oil on the turkey breast. Season both sides with salt and turkey seasoning, then rub the remaining half tablespoon of oil over the side of the skin.

2. Preheat the 350°F air fryer and cook skin-side down for 20 minutes, flip and cook until the internal temperature is 160°F using an instant read thermometer for an additional 30 to 40 minutes, depending on your breast size. Let stand 10 minutes before carving.

Nutritional Information

- Calories: 226
- Carbohydrates: 0g
- Fat: 10g
- Protein: 32.5g
- Sugar: 0g
- Cholesterol: 84mg

Air Fryer Cookbook

Hot Rosemary Pickled Chicken

• Servings: 2 • Preparation time: 1h • Cook time: 30 minutes •

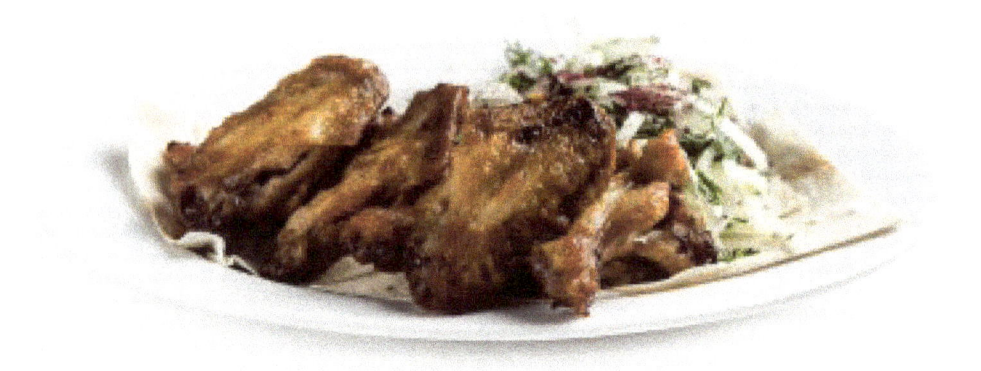

HOT CHICKEN

Ingredients

For the brine:
- 2 ½ cups warm water
- ¼ cup salt
- ¼ cup sugar
- 1 pound chicken

For the marinade:
- 1 ½ cups nonfat yogurt
- ¼ cup rosemary
- ½ tbsp ground cloves
- 2 cloves
- Garlic
- 2 tbsp lemon juice
- ½ tsp salt
- ¼ tsp black pepper

Steps to Cook

Brine the chicken:

1. In a large bowl, put water, salt, and sugar. Whisk until the salt and sugar dissolve. Add the chicken and soak for 30 minutes. Remove, rinse and dry. Let stand in the refrigerator for a couple of hours.

Prepare the marinade:

2. In a medium bowl, put all the ingredients for the marinade. Rub evenly over each surface of the chicken.

3. Preheat the air fryer to 350°F. Spray the fryer basket with kitchen spray. Put the chicken in the fryer and cook 30 minutes. Turn chicken over and cook another 30 minutes or until fully cooked. The skin should be crisp.

Nutritional Information

- Calories: 301
- Carbohydrates: 0g
- Fat: 18g
- Protein: 36g
- Sugar: 0g
- Cholesterol: 190mg

Grilled Cheese With Mayonnaise

• Servings: 1 • Preparation time: 5minutes • Cook time: 12 minutes •

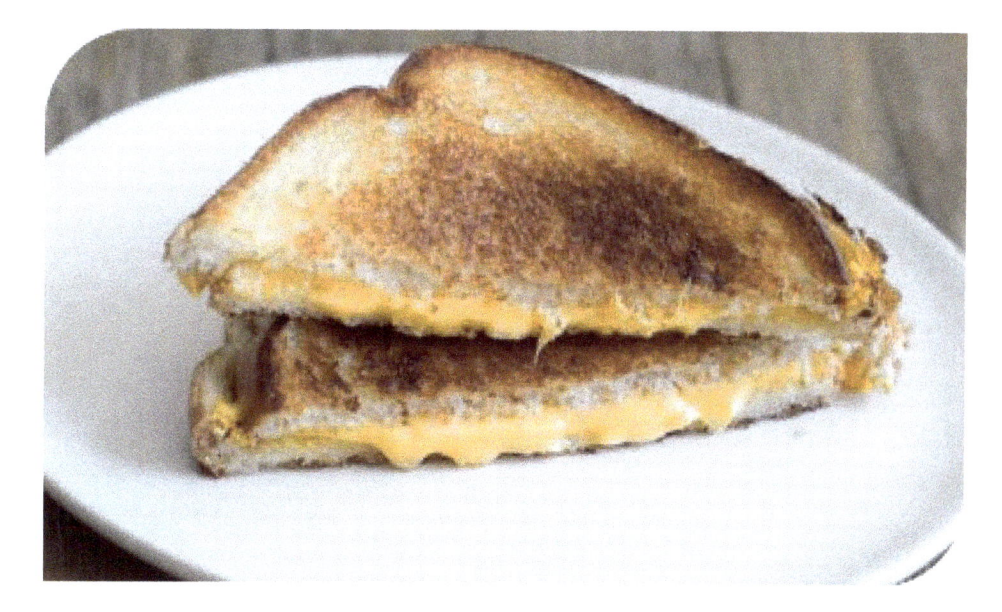

GRILLED

Ingredients

- 2 slices of bread
- 2 teaspoons of butter or kitchen spray
- 2 slices of cheese
- ¼ pear, thinly sliced

Steps to Cook

1. Preheat the air fryer to 180ºC.

2. Butter one side of each slice of bread, making sure all the bread is covered.

3. Add cheese and pear. Fold the cheese slices between the bread slices making sure no cheese comes out of the bread slices.

4. Add to the fryer and cook for 8 minutes before turning and cooking for another 3-4 minutes on the second side.

....

Nutritional Information

- Calories: 473
- Carbohydrates: 35g
- Fat: 28g
- Protein: 20g
- Sugar: 8g
- Cholesterol: 80mg

Canned Mussel Pie

• Servings: 2 • Preparation time: 5 minutes • Cook time: 20-25 minutes •

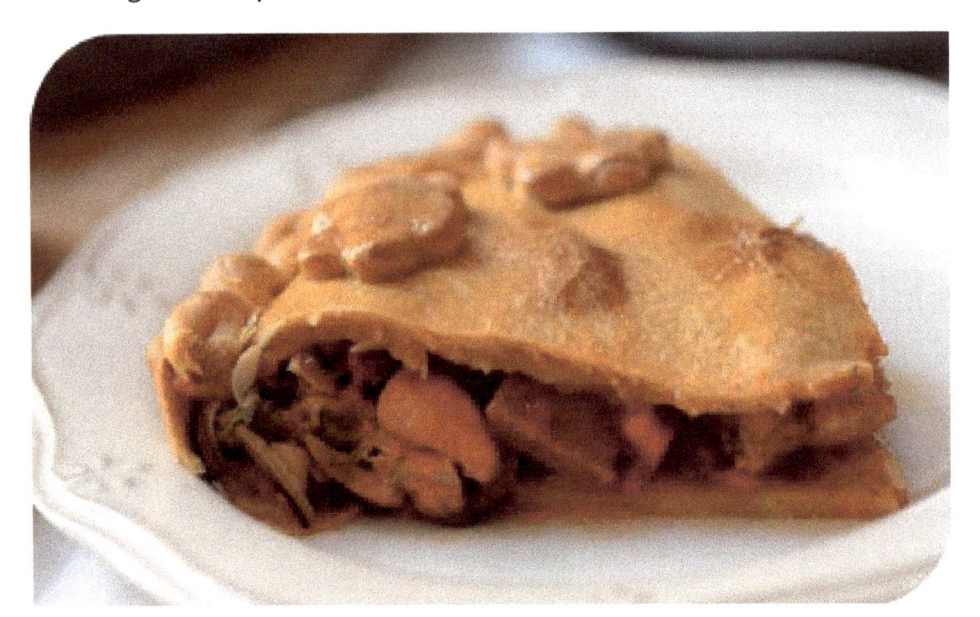

DELICIOUS

Ingredients

- 1 fresh empanada dough
- 2 cans mussels in brine
- 1 medium onion
- 1 leek
- ¼ red pepper
- Bacon in small pieces
- 1 egg
- Oil and salt

Steps to Cook

1. Chop the onion, the leek, the pepper and fry in a pan with oil.

2. When you see that the vegetables are done, add the pieces of bacon and the chopped mussels. Make two turns and remove from the fire.

3. Drain the oil well and let it warm.

4. Stretch the dough and distribute the farce in half of it, cover on top with the other half and join the edges.

5. Paint with beaten egg and make a small cut in the center, so that it breathes through it.

6. Take to air fryer, preheated to 200ºC, and leave until it does not brown, about 20/25 minutes approximately.

Nutritional Information

- Calories: 615
- Carbohydrates: 63g
- Fat: 31g
- Protein: 11g
- Sugar: 3g
- Cholesterol: 300mg

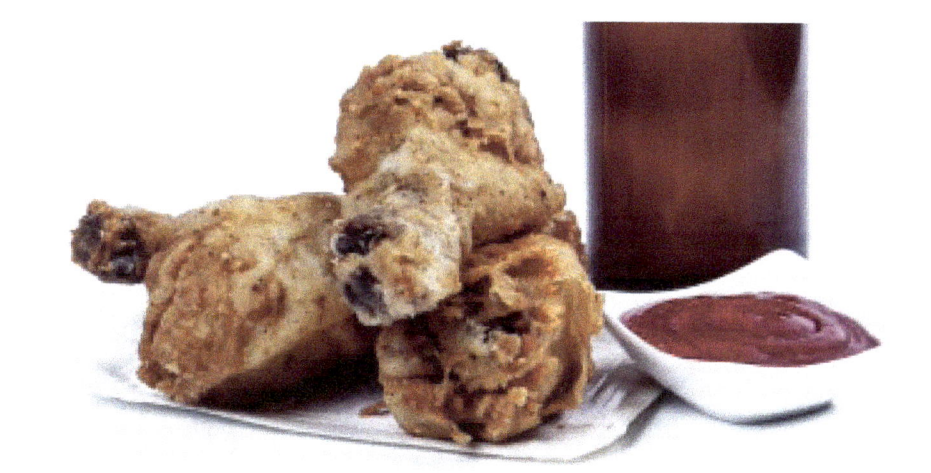

TASTEFUL

Crispy Chicken Fried in Beer

• Servings: 6 • Preparation time: 45 minutes• Cook time: 20 minutes •

Ingredients

Source #1:

- 3 cups all-purpose flour
- 2 tbsp of table salt
- 2 tbsp freshly ground pepper
- 1 tsp of cayenne
- 2 tsp of paprika
- 1 ½ tsp garlic powder
- 1 ½ tsp onion powder

Source #2:

- 1 ⅓ cups all-purpose flour
- 1 ⅓ cups of beer
- 1 teaspoon salt
- ¼ tsp ground black pepper
- 2 beaten eggs

Frying:

- Vegetable oil for frying
- 3 lbs of chicken thighs and/or breasts

Steps to Cook

Breaded:

1. Add all the ingredients defined for the Source #1 and mix.

2. Repeat the process with the ingredients defined for the Source #2.

3. Check the consistency of the mixture with beer and adjust the texture as necessary.

4. Working in batches, bread the chicken in the Source #1 (flour and condiments), then in the Source #2 (beer batter) and finally again in the Source #1, shaking the pieces to remove the excess each time.

Frying:

5. Preheat the air fryer to 350 ° F (177 ° C) for 20 minutes. Add the chicken pieces in a single layer, working in batches as needed and turning the chicken over to ensure even cooking.

6. If it is not ready, cook for 15 minutes.

Nutritional Information

- Calories: 548
- Carbohydrates: 9g
- Fat: 24g
- Protein: 66g
- Sugar: 0g
- Cholesterol: 83mg

Air Fryer Cookbook

Cheese Pay with Cookie

• Servings: 2 • Preparation time: 5 minutes • Cook time: 25 minutes •

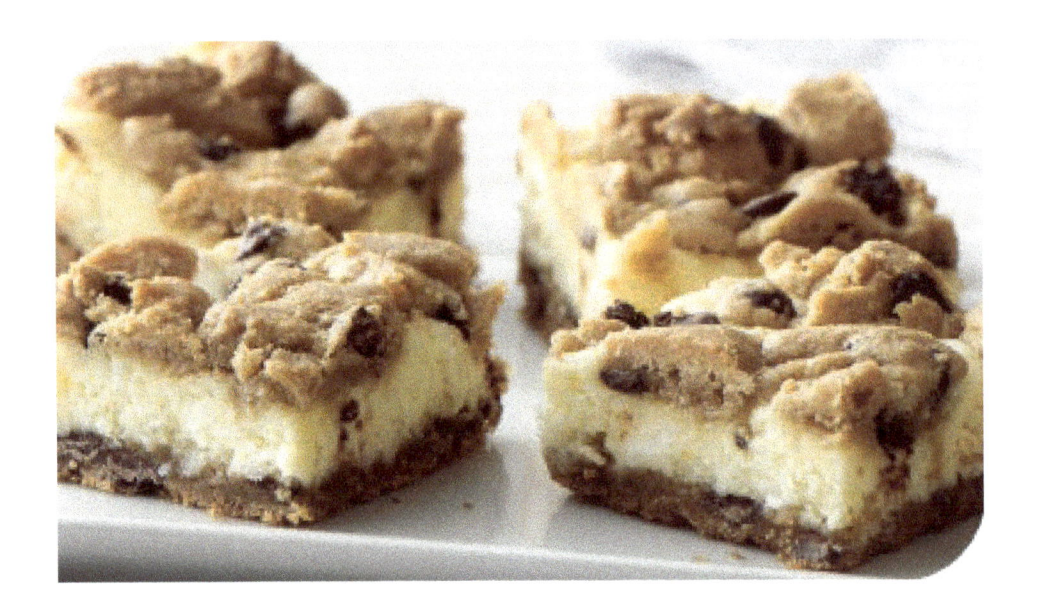

CREAMY

Ingredients

- 1 package of Maria cookie, 170 g
- ½ cups butter, melted
- 1 can of condensed milk
- 1 can of evaporated milk
- 3 eggs
- 7 oz. of cream cheese

Steps to Cook

1. Preheat the air fryer to 160°C.

2. Grind the cookies, reserve a little of the cookie to cover the pie and leave a golden crust.

3. Mix the rest of the cookies with the butter to form a paste and place in the base of the pie pan. Reserve.

4. Blend the remaining ingredients. Empty the mixture into the mold and sprinkle the cookie that you reserved on top.

5. Put into air fryer and cover with aluminum foil for 30 minutes or until firm.

6. Chill and refrigerate 2 hours before serving.

Nutritional Information

- Calories: 108
- Carbohydrates: 12g
- Fat: 6g
- Protein: 1g
- Sugar: 5g
- Cholesterol: 279mg

Spicy Potatoes

• Servings:4 • Preparation time: 5 minutes • Cook time: 20 minutes •

SPICY

Ingredients

Ingredients for the potatoes:

- 2 large potatoes
- olive oil
- salt

Ingredients for sauce:

- 1 onion
- 1 clove Garlic
- 1 glass of crushed natural tomato
- 1 pinch saffron
- 1 tsp sugar
- 2 to 3 Cayenne Peppers
- 1 point ham
- 1 tsp hot paprika
- 1 tsp of food coloring,
- 1 tbsp of flour
- 1 splash of sherry vinegar
- 1 tbsp of olive oil
- Salt

Steps to Cook

1. Peel the potatoes and cut into cubes of about 2 or 3 cm each, pass through water and dry very well.

2. Sprinkle the potatoes with oil and preheat the Air fryer for a few minutes at 180ºC.

3. Subsequently, place the potatoes in the basket and set the timer for about 20 minutes at 180ºC.

4. Shake the potatoes from time to time. Salt and reserve.

5. Prepare the sauce:

6. Finely chop the onion together with the garlic clove and sauté in the oil over low heat.

7. Add the ham tip and two or three cayenne peppers.

8. When the onion is transparent add the hot paprika and the saffron threads, turn around and add the crushed tomato.

9. Season together with the teaspoon of sugar and leave to cook, stirring for 5 minutes.

10. Incorporate the flour diluted in water, mix, cover with water, add the dye and cook for 15 min. plus.

11. At the end of cooking add the vinegar drizzle, mix well, remove the ham tip and pass the

12. rest of ingredients through the mixer.

13. Strain into the Chinese and it is ready.

Nutritional Information

- Calories: 269
- Carbohydrates: 32g
- Fat: 1g
- Protein: 5.1g
- Sugar: 3.6g
- Cholesterol: 0mg

Air Fryer Cookbook

Grilled Provolons

• Servings: 4 • Preparation time: 5 minutes • Cook time: 20 minutes •

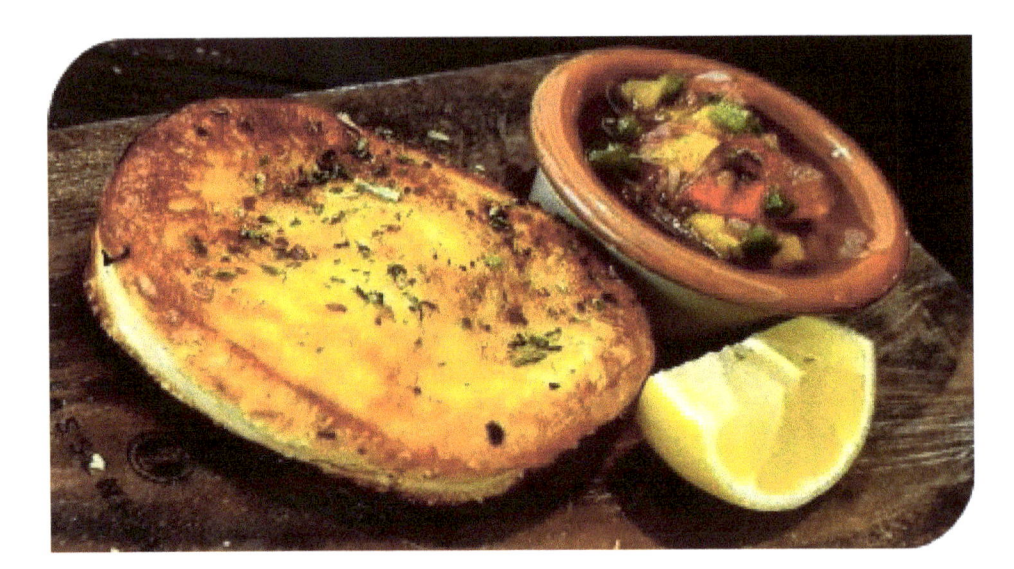

BUDGET FRIENDLY

Ingredients

- A slice of Provolone cheese
- 1 ripe red tomato
- 1 aubergine
- 1 zucchini
- 1 onion
- 1 red pepper
- Salt

Steps to Cook

1. Preheat the Air fryer for a few minutes at 180ºC.

2. Put the separator on the Air fryer and distribute the eggplant on one side and the zucchini on the other, cook for 15 minutes at 180ºC. Once finished, remove and correct the salt. Then do the same with the onion and pepper. Reserve next to the rest of the vegetables. Place some tomato slices in the bottom of a clay pot and place in the Air fryer basket for 3 minutes at 180ºC temperature. Then add the Provolone cheese, sprinkling on top with a little oregano

3. Set the timer for about 8 minutes at 180ºC.

4. When the cheese is melted and golden, put on the plate and surround with the grill of vegetables.

Nutritional Information

- Calories: 245
- Carbohydrates: 8g
- Fat: 17g
- Protein: 15g
- Sugar: 2g
- Cholesterol: 84mg

Typical Rice from Valencia

• Servings: 2 • Preparation time: 10 minutes • Cook time: 60 minutes •

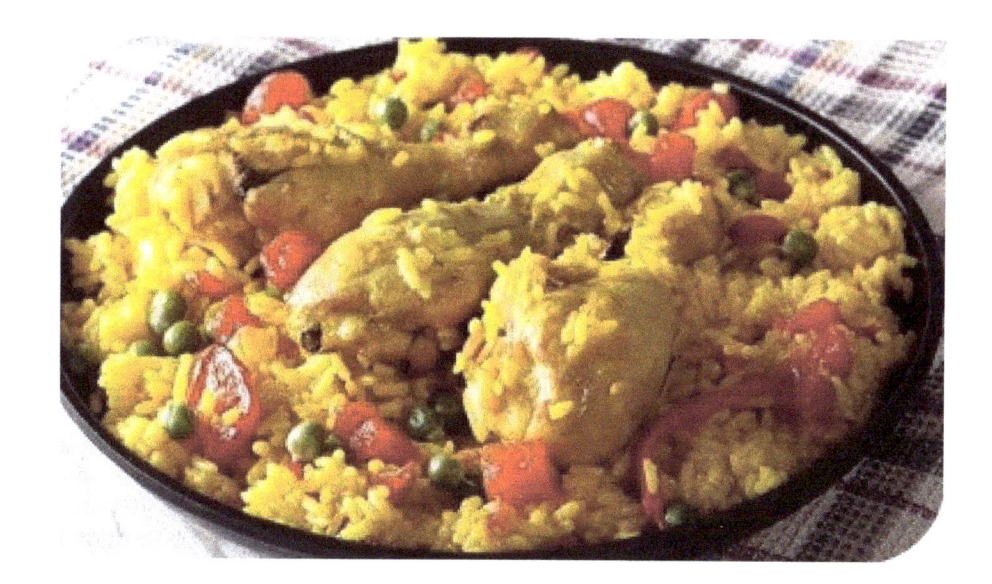

EXUBARANT

Ingredients

- 50 g cooked chickpeas
- ½ lb of chicken
- 100 g turnip
- 1 medium tomato
- 1 head garlic
- 2 cups of rice
- Saffron
- oil
- Salt
- Water
- Olive oil

Steps to Cook

1. In a saucepan, with a little oil, fry the chicken and add the chopped turnip. Once golden add water (1 ½ cup), when it begins to boil add the chickpeas, saffron, salt and cook for 30 minutes.

2. In a clay pot place the rice, the tomato cut in two, the garlic head and the ingredients that you have used to make the broth (rib, turnip and chickpeas). Then add the broth to cook, twice the broth than rice.

3. Preheat the Air fryer for a few minutes at 200ºC.

4. Place the clay pot in the basket of the Air fryer and set the timer about 45 minutes at 200ºC temperature.

Nutritional Information

- Calories: 707
- Carbohydrates: 55g
- Fat: 43g
- Protein: 25g
- Sugar: 5g
- Cholesterol: 83mg

Eggplants Stuffed With Cod

• Servings: 4 • Preparation time: 10 minutes • Cook time: 15 minutes •

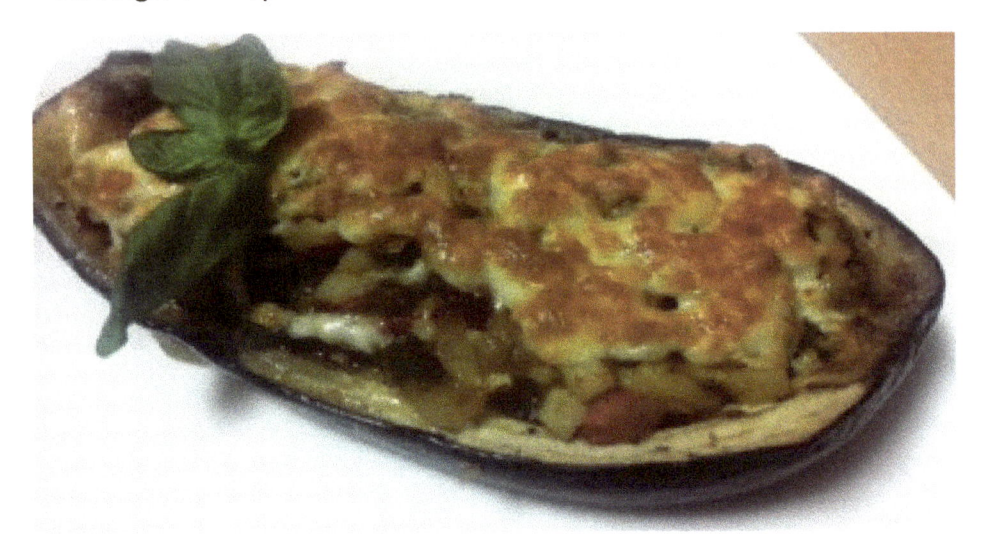

TASTEFUL

Ingredients

- 4 aubergines
- 7 oz. of crumbled cod
- 3 ½ oz. of camembert cheese
- Salt and pepper
- 1 ½ oz. grated cheese for gratin
- Salt

Steps to Cook

1. Cut the eggplants in half and empty, reserving the pulp.

2. Cut the cheese into small cubes and set aside.

3. Mix the pulp of the aubergines with the cheese cubes and the cod, previously desalted. Salt grinding.

4. Fill the aubergines with the mixture, squeezing a little so that they fill well.

5. Preheat the Air fryer for a few minutes at 180°C and once ready distribute the aubergines stuffed in the basket of the Air fryer. Set the timer for about 15 minutes at 180°C.

6. At the end of the time, open the Air fryer and sprinkle with the grated cheese.

7. Reprogram the timer for another 5 minutes at 180°C.

Nutritional Information

- Calories: 198
- Carbohydrates: 8g
- Fat: 10g
- Protein: 19g
- Sugar: 4g
- Cholesterol: 60mg

Leek Quiche

• Servings:8 • Preparation time: 10 minutes • Cook time: 20 minutes •

Ingredients

- 4 Leeks well washed and cut
- 1 onion
- 1 terrine of ½ lb of cheese
- cool Quark type
- 4 tbsp of grated cheese
- 4 eggs
- 2 tbsp of
- olive oil
- Salt and pepper
- 1 shortcrust pastry dough

Steps to Cook

1. Wash the leeks and chop the white part.

2. Cut the onion and chop. Poach the leeks together with the onion, in a pan with a little oil.

3. Season and cover, if all the oil is absorbed add a little water and finish poaching. When the leeks is ready reserve. Meanwhile, in a separate bowl add the eggs and beat, add the fresh cheese and mix until obtaining a homogeneous cream. Then salt and incorporate the grated cheese.

4. Arrange the breeze dough on a container and prick with a fork to prevent it from swelling. Deposit the poached vegetables on top, distributing them well and incorporate the preparation of the eggs and other ingredients

5. Preheat the Air fryer a few minutes to 180ºC.

6. Put the container in the basket of the Air fryer and set the timer about 25 minutes to 180ºC.

7. If everything does not fit in the same container, you can do it in two phases.

Nutritional Information

- Calories: 260
- Carbohydrates: 23g
- Fat: 12g
- Protein: 16g
- Sugar: 1g
- Cholesterol: 45mg

Mushrooms With Ham

• Servings: 4 • Preparation time: 5 minutes • Cook time: 10 minutes •

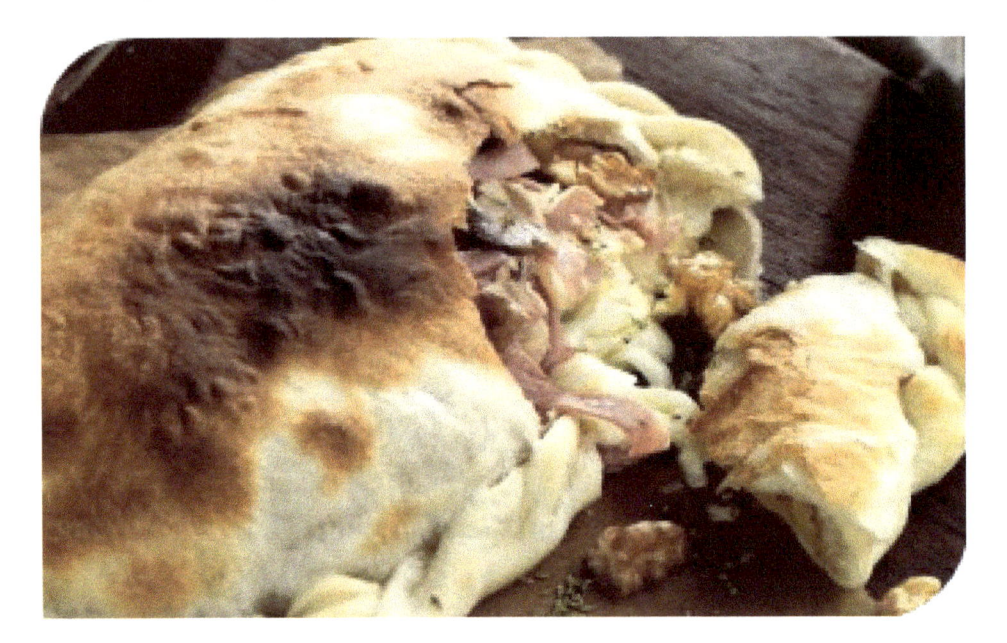

CRISPY

Ingredients

- 5 oz. of cultivated mushrooms
- 1 small brick of cream for cooking
- 3 ½ oz. of Serrano ham
- ½ lb of shortcrust pastry
- Salt
- Pepper

Steps to Cook

1. Cut the mushrooms and ham into small pieces. Then mix in a bowl with the cream and season with salt and pepper.

2. Divide and cut the shortcrust pastry into eight squares of 10 cm each. Fill the center of each square with a tablespoon of the previous mixture.

3. To close the sachets, join each corner of the square to the center, then prick the dough a little and paint with beaten egg.

4. Preheat the Air fryer a few minutes to 200ºC.

5. Place the sachets in the basket of the Air fryer and set the timer for about 15 minutes at 200ºC temperature.

Nutritional Information

- Calories: 227
- Carbohydrates: 16g
- Fat: 15gg
- Protein: 7g
- Sugar: 10g
- Cholesterol: 49mg

Monkfish Skewers

• Servings: 4 • Preparation time: 5 minutes • Cook time: 5 minutes •

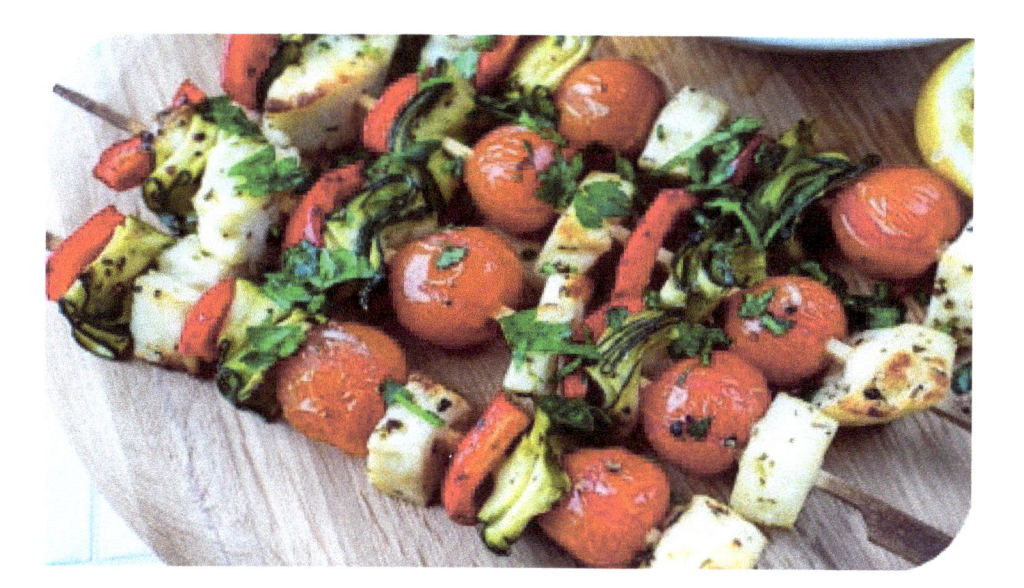

FLAVORSOME

Ingredients

- ½ lb monkfish
- ½ lb cherry tomatoes
- 1 zucchini
- 4 mushrooms
- 1 green pepper
- 1 tbsp of olive oil
- Salt
- Chopsticks

Steps to Cook

1. Assemble the skewers interspersing Cherry tomato, monkfish, zucchini, mushroom, pepper, until completing the toothpick or skewer as seen in the photo.

2. Preheat the Air fryer for a few minutes at 180ºC.

3. Meanwhile, brush the skewers with a little oil.

4. Put them in the basket and set the timer for about 5 minutes at 180ºC temperature.

5. Turn around when they are a little golden.

6. Finish browning and serving.

Nutritional Information

- Calories: 97
- Carbohydrates: 14g
- Fat: 1g
- Protein: 18g
- Sugar: 10g
- Cholesterol: 17mg

Air Fryer Cookbook

Sirloin With Vegetables

• Servings: 4 • Preparation time: 5 minutes • Cook time: 30 minutes •

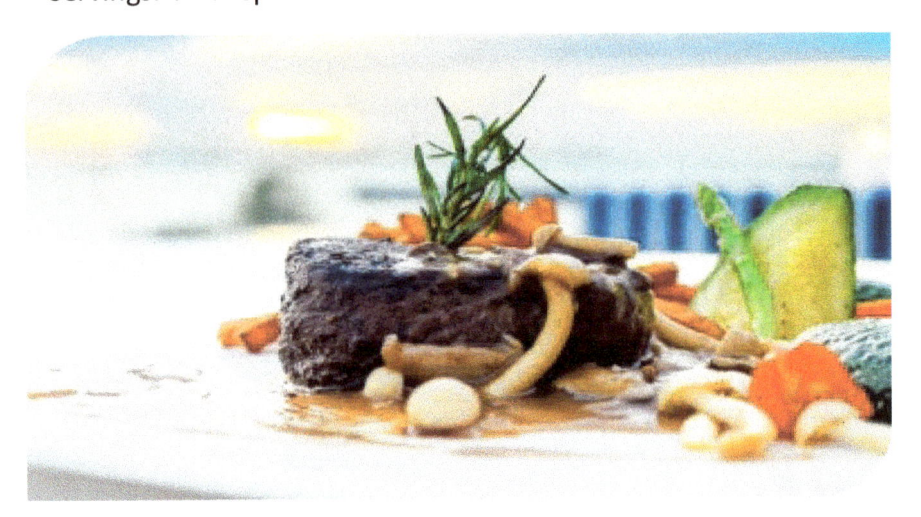

HEALTHY

Ingredients

- 1 lb beef sirloin
- 1 carrot
- 1 onion
- 1 broccoli
- 1 pepper
- Soy sauce

Steps to Cook

1. Clean the sirloin and cut into 5 cm cubes and set aside. Wash the vegetables and cut into cubes or the way you want.

2. Preheat the Air fryer for a few minutes at 180ºC.

3. Put a container in the basket of the Air fryer with a little water, add the vegetables with salt and pepper and set the timer for about 30 minutes at 180ºC.

4. When the vegetables are punctured when crispy, add the meat and a good stream of soy sauce.

5. Let cook about 15 minutes more.

6. Remove the container from the Air fryer and strain all the juice that was made by cooking the meat with the vegetables and soy sauce.

7. In a separate saucepan, reduce the sauce to the fire for 5 minutes and add again to the meat with vegetables.

8. Serve in a dish accompanied by rice, couscous or quinoa.

Nutritional Information

- Calories: 189
- Carbohydrates: 7g
- Fat: 5g
- Protein: 49g
- Sugar: 2g
- Cholesterol: 92mg

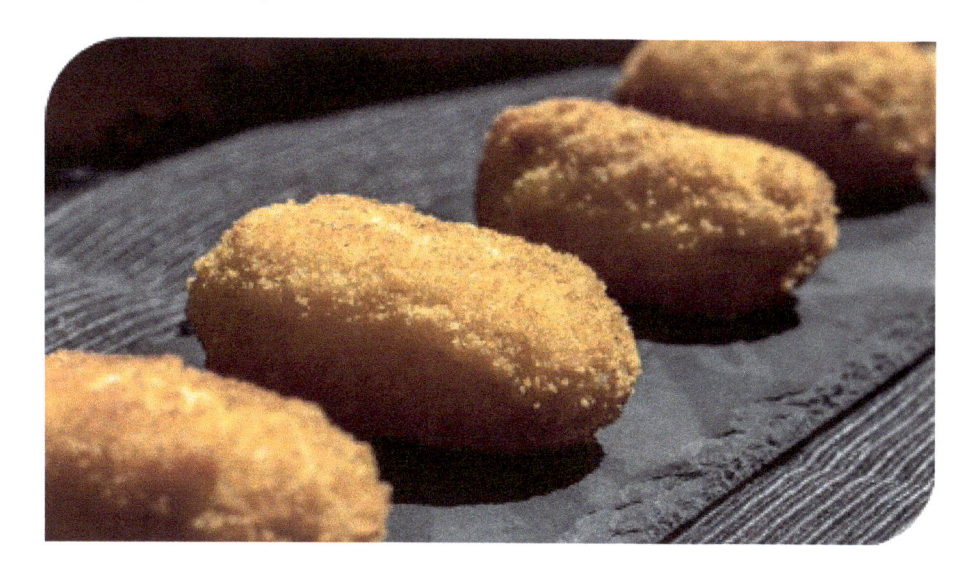

DELICIOUS

Homemade Croquettes

• Servings: 4 • Preparation time: 15 minutes • Cook time: 60 minutes •

Ingredients

• Cooked meat without skin: ham, chicken, chorizo.

• ½ onion

• Extra virgin olive oil

• Salt

• Pepper

• 2 tbsp of flour

For the bechamel:

• 2 butter spoons

• 3 cups skim milk

• Nutmeg

For the batter:

• Bread crumbs

• 2 eggs

• Salt

Steps to Cook

1. Finely chop the onion and sauté in a pan with extra virgin olive oil. Then add 2 tbsp of flour and 2 tablespoons of margarine.

2. Stir slowly and gradually add the milk (previously hot), without stopping stirring. Add a pinch of nutmeg and salt. Mix until you get a creamy consistency, add the meat of the stew and a pinch of salt.

3. Once a homogeneous paste is achieved, leave to cool in the refrigerator for about 2 hours.

4. Then shape the croquettes, go through beaten egg, flour and breadcrumbs.

5. While preheating the Air fryer for a few minutes at 180ºC.

6. Put the kibbles in the basket of the Air fryer and set the timer for 15 minutes at 180ºC.

7. Make the croquettes in batches

Nutritional Information

• Calories: 58

• Carbohydrates: 6g

• Fat: 2g

• Protein: 4g

• Sugar: 4g

• Cholesterol: 19mg

Tuna Empanada

• Servings: 4 • Preparation time: 5 minutes • Cook time: 30 minutes •

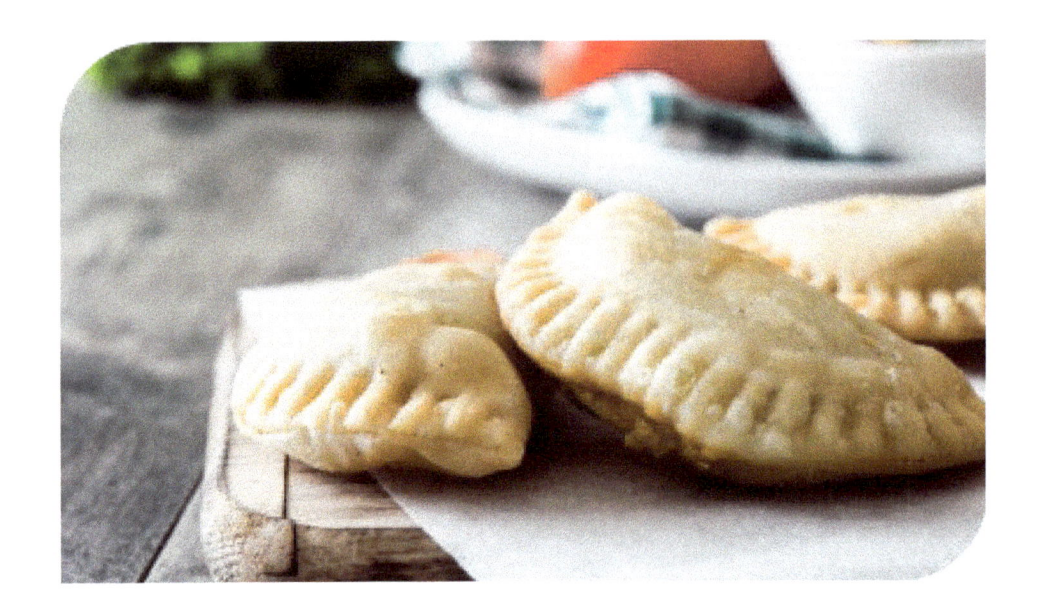

HIGH CALORIE

Ingredients

- 2 boiled eggs
- 2 cans of tuna
- 1 cup fried tomato.
- 1 sheet of broken dough.

Steps to Cook

1. Cut the eggs into cubes and mix with the tuna and tomato.
2. Roll out the sheet of shortcrust pastry and cut into two equal squares.
3. Put the tuna, eggs and tomato mixture on one of the squares.
4. Cover with the other, join at the ends and decorate with leftover bits.
5. Preheat the Air fryer for a few minutes at 180°C.
6. Put in the basket of the Air fryer and set the timer 15 minutes to 180°C.

Nutritional Information

- Calories: 460
- Carbohydrates: 32g
- Fat: 28g
- Protein: 20g
- Sugar: 3g
- Cholesterol: 166mg

Scrambled Egg

• Servings: 1 • Preparation time: 5 minutes • Cook time: 20 minutes •

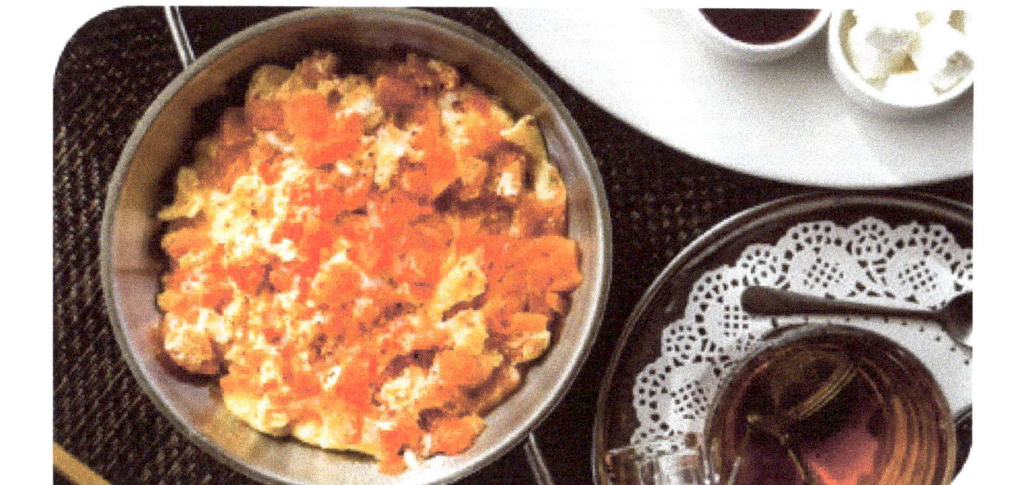

AMAZINGLY DELICIOUS

Ingredients

- 2 eggs
- 1 tablespoon of tomato sauce
- 1 good handful of frozen peas
- 1 slice of sobrasada cut into pieces
- 1 splash of olive oil
- salt and pepper

Steps to Cook

1. Preheat the Air fryer for about 3 minutes at 180ºC.

2. Lightly brush the clay pot with the oil.

3. Spread the tomato sauce over the base of the casserole and place the peas on top.

4. Crack the two eggs and carefully place them on the pea bed.

5. Spread the sobrasada pieces around the eggs and season to taste.

6. Put the casserole in the basket, close and set the timer for about 12 minutes at 180ºC.

7. Take out the casserole very carefully so as not to get burned and serve in the same container.

Nutritional Information

- Calories: 304
- Carbohydrates: 4g
- Fat: 24g
- Protein: 18g
- Sugar: 10g
- Cholesterol: 415mg

Air Fryer Cookbook

Eggs with Potatoes and Ham

• Servings: 2 • Preparation time: 5 minutes • Cook time: 15 minutes •

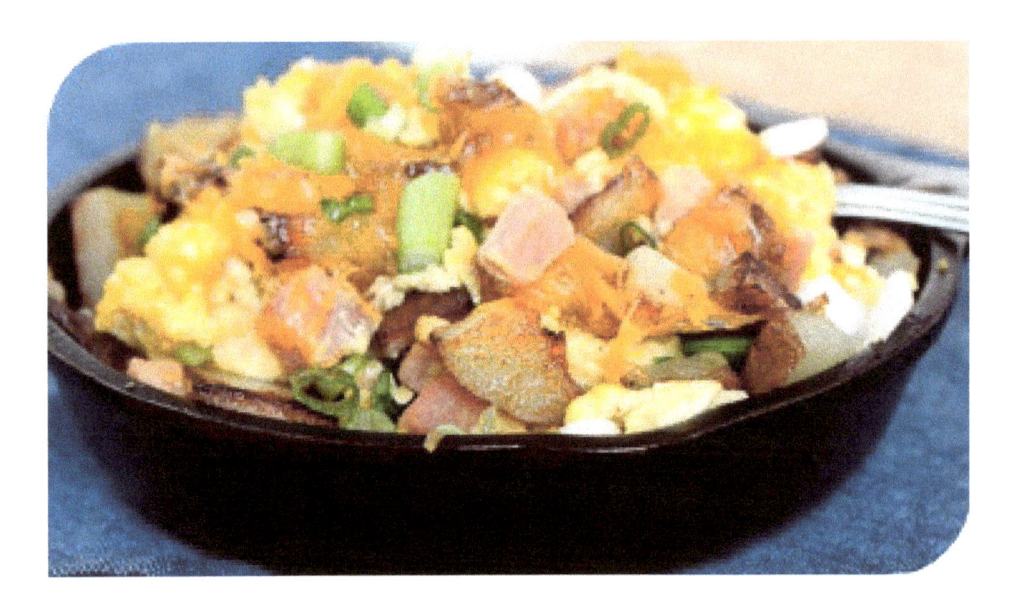

BEAUTIFUL

Ingredients

- 1 ½ lb of potatoes
- Salt
- 1 tbsp of olive oil
- ¼ lb of Iberico Ham
- 4 eggs

Steps to Cook

1. Cut the French fries elongated, go through plenty of water and dry well with kitchen paper.

2. Spray with oil and preheat the Air fryer for a few minutes at 200ºC. Put the potatoes in the basket of the Air fryer and set the timer for 25 minutes at 200ºC. When we see that they are beginning to turn golden, put vegetable paper under the potatoes and add the eggs.

3. Put it back in the Air fryer for 5 more minutes.

4. Finally add Iberian Ham flakes.

5. If you want to go faster while the potatoes are fried in the Air fryer, you can prepare the grilled eggs in a small pan and then mix with the potatoes and ham on the plate.

Nutritional Information

- Calories: 250
- Carbohydrates: 23g
- Fat: 10g
- Protein: 17g
- Sugar: 2g
- Cholesterol: 217mg

Classic Flamenquins

• Servings: 4 • Preparation time: 10 minutes • Cook time: 20 minutes •

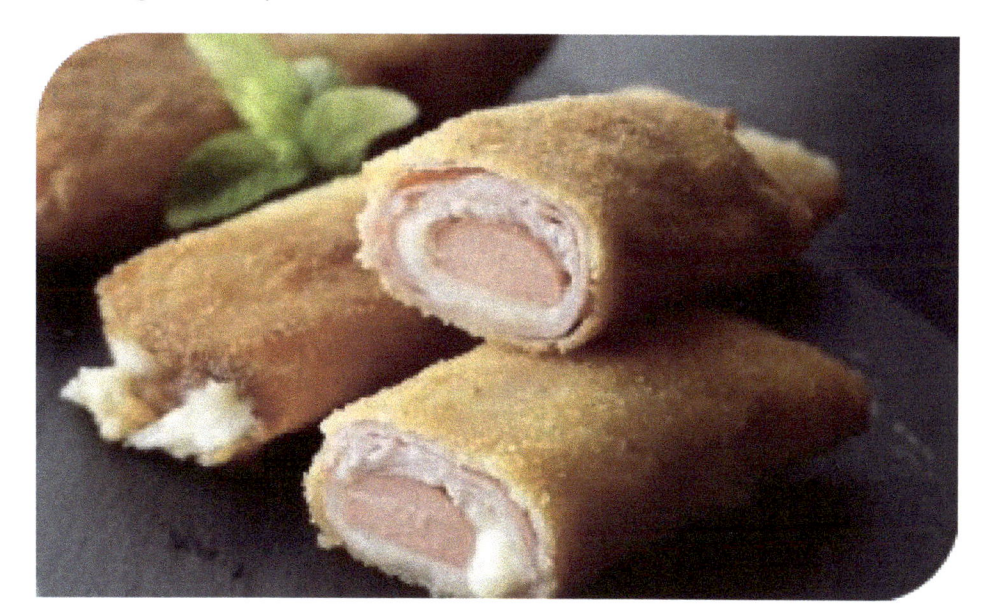

DELICIOUS

Ingredients

- ½ lb of very thin cut pork fillets
- 2 boiled and chopped eggs
- ¼ lb minced serrano ham
- 1 beaten egg
- Bread crumbs

Steps to Cook

1. Make a roll with the pork fillets, introduce half a cooked egg and the Serrano ham inside. So that the roll does not lose its shape, hold it with a string or chopsticks.

2. Pass the rolls through beaten egg and then through the breadcrumbs until a good layer is formed.

3. Preheat the Air fryer for a few minutes at 180ºC.

4. Put the rolls in the basket and program the timer for about 8 minutes at 180ºC.

5. Serve right away

Nutritional Information

- Calories: 269
- Carbohydrates: 12g
- Fat: 13g
- Protein: 26g
- Sugar: 2g
- Cholesterol: 204mg

Air Fryer Cookbook

Breaded Chicken Fillets

• Servings: 4 • Preparation time: 5 minutes • Cook time: 15 minutes •

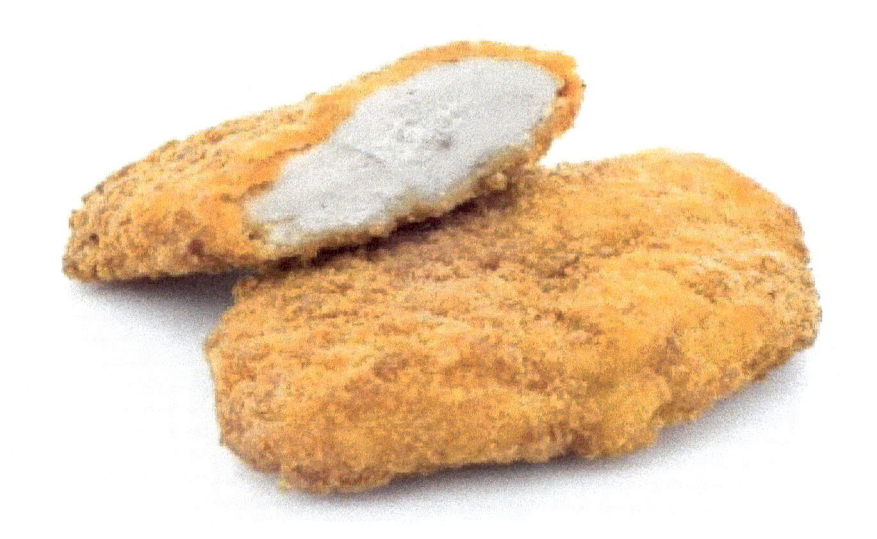

YUMMY

Ingredients

- 1 lb chicken fillets (breasts)
- 1 egg
- Parsley
- Garlic
- Salt
- Olive oil
- Flour

Steps to Cook

1. Cut the fillets thin and season with salt and pepper.

2. Go through flour, beaten egg (already mixed with parsley and garlic) and finally go through breadcrumbs.

3. Spray with oil and preheat the Air fryer for a few minutes at 180ºC.

4. Put the fillets in the basket of the Air fryer and set the timer 15 minutes at 180ºC.

Nutritional Information

- Calories: 219
- Carbohydrates: 14g
- Fat: 7g
- Protein: 25g
- Sugar: 1g
- Cholesterol: 113mg

Baked Hasselback Potatoes

• Servings: 4 • Preparation time: 3 minutes• Cook time: 40 minutes •

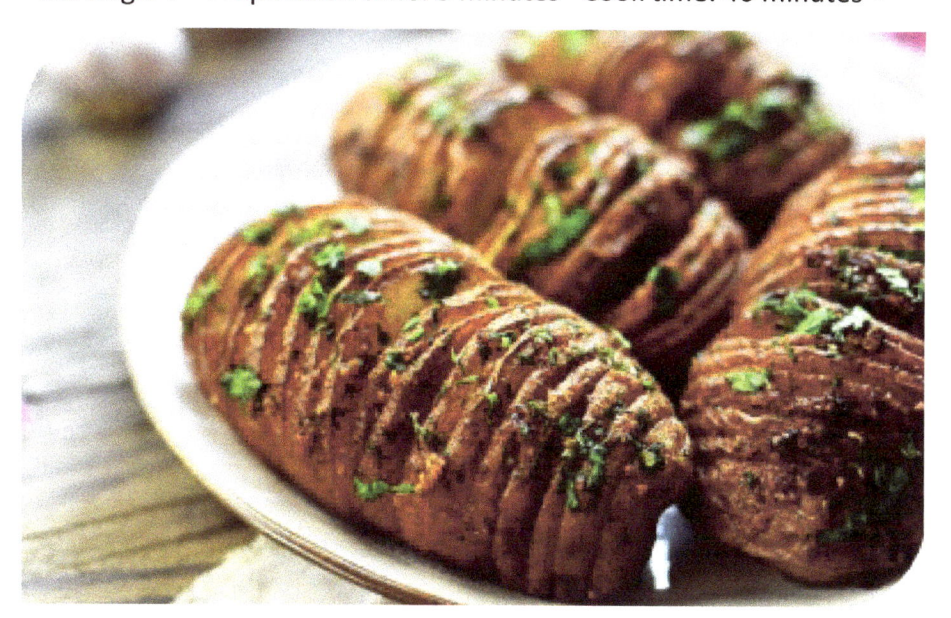

Ingredients

- 4 medium reddish potatoes washed and drained
- 6 tsp olive oil
- 2 ½ tsp of salt
- ¼ tsp black pepper
- ¼ tsp garlic powder
- 1 oz. of melted butter
- 1 ½ tsp of parsley, freshly chopped, to decorate

Steps to Cook

1. Wash and scrub the potatoes. Let them dry with a paper towel.

2. Cut the slits 6mm apart on the potatoes, stopping before you cut it completely, so that all the slices are connected about 13mm at the bottom of the potato.

3. Select Preheat on the air fryer, set it to 175°C.

4. Cover the potatoes with olive oil and season evenly with salt, black pepper and garlic powder.

5. Add the potatoes in the air fryer and cook for 30 minutes at 175°C.

6. Brush the melted butter over the potatoes and cook for another 10 minutes at 175°C.

7. Garnish with Freshly Chopped Parsley

Nutritional Information

- Calories: 105
- Carbohydrates: 21g
- Fat: 2g
- Protein: 2g
- Sugar: 1g
- Cholesterol: 300m

Air Fryer Cookbook

Fish Cake For Lunch

• Servings: 4 • Preparation time: 5 minutes • Cook time: 15 minutes •

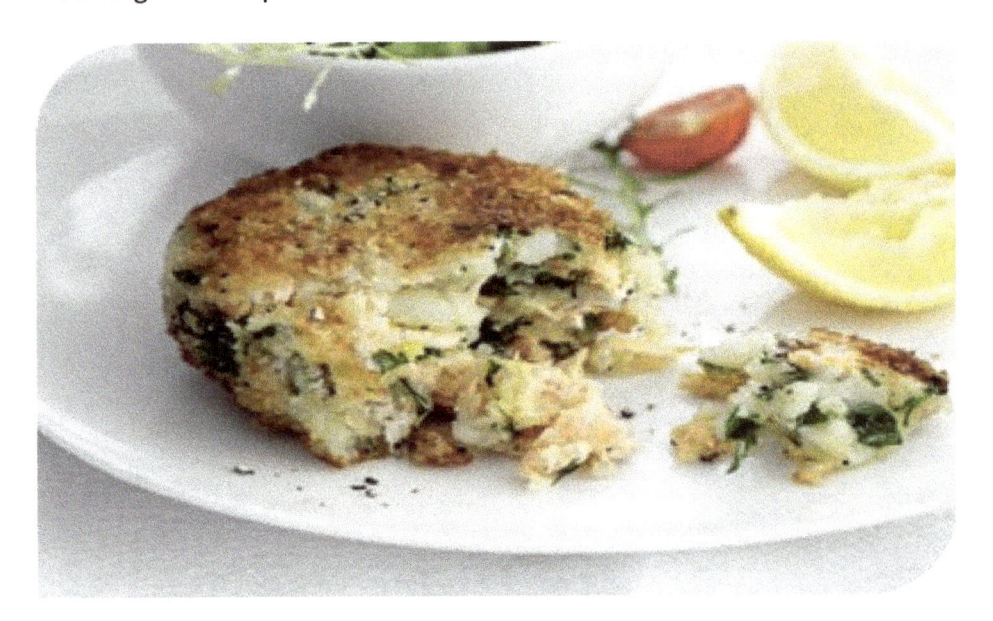

DELIGHTFUL

Ingredients

- 7 oz. monkfish or hake
- 1 cup cream
- ½ cup fried tomato
- 4 eggs
- Salt and pepper

Steps to Cook

1. Mix all the ingredients except the eggs.
2. With a blender crush everything very well.
3. Once a paste is formed, add the eggs one by one.
4. Mix well and place in a bowl smeared with oil.
5. Cover with aluminum foil.
6. Preheat the Air fryer a few minutes to 180ºC.
7. Put the container with the cake in the basket of the Air fryer.
8. Set the timer for 30 minutes at 180ºC.
9. Once tempered, unmold and cut

Nutritional Information

- Calories: 229
- Carbohydrates: 3g
- Fat: 17g
- Protein: 16g
- Sugar: 3g
- Cholesterol: 244mg

Salmon Wrapped

• Servings: 1 • Preparation time: 5 minutes • Cook time: 15 minutes •

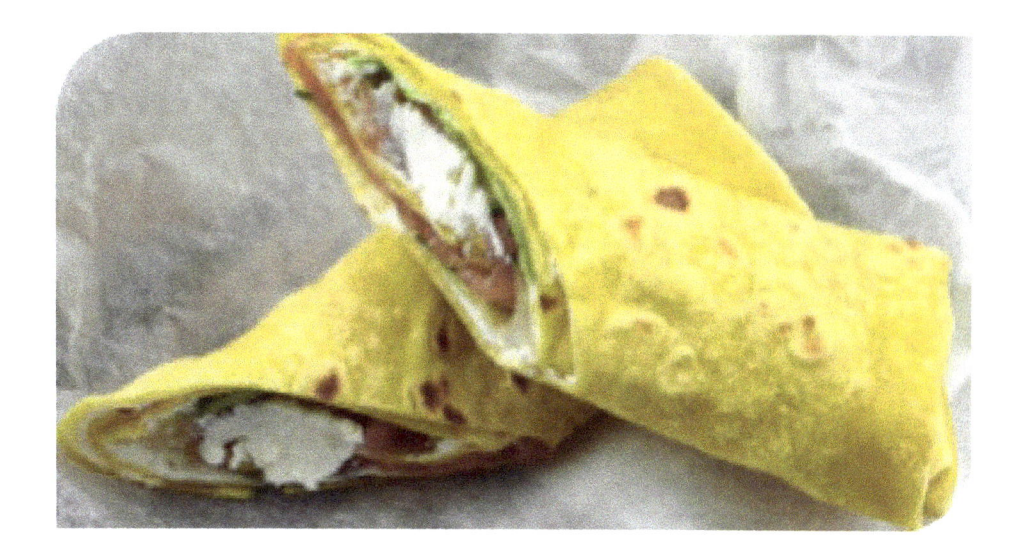

DELICIOUS

Ingredients

- 4 ½ oz. salmon
- Edged dough
- Dill
- Lemon
- Salt and pepper

Steps to Cook

1. Sprinkle the salmon with a few drops of lemon juice, season with salt and pepper and add the dill.

2. Arrange each salmon loin on top of a phyllo sheet. Wrap the salmon and brush with olive oil or beaten egg.

3. Preheat the Air fryer for a few minutes at 180ºC.

4. Put the salmon packages in the basket of the Air fryer and set the timer for 10 to 15 minutes at 180ºC, depending on the thickness of the salmon.

5. Serve accompanied with soy sauce and a refreshing salad

Nutritional Information

- Calories: 303
- Carbohydrates: 6g
- Fat: 19g
- Protein: 27g
- Sugar: 2g
- Cholesterol: 73mg

Greek-Style Potatoes

• Servings: 4 • Preparation time: 30 minutes • Cook time: 28 minutes •

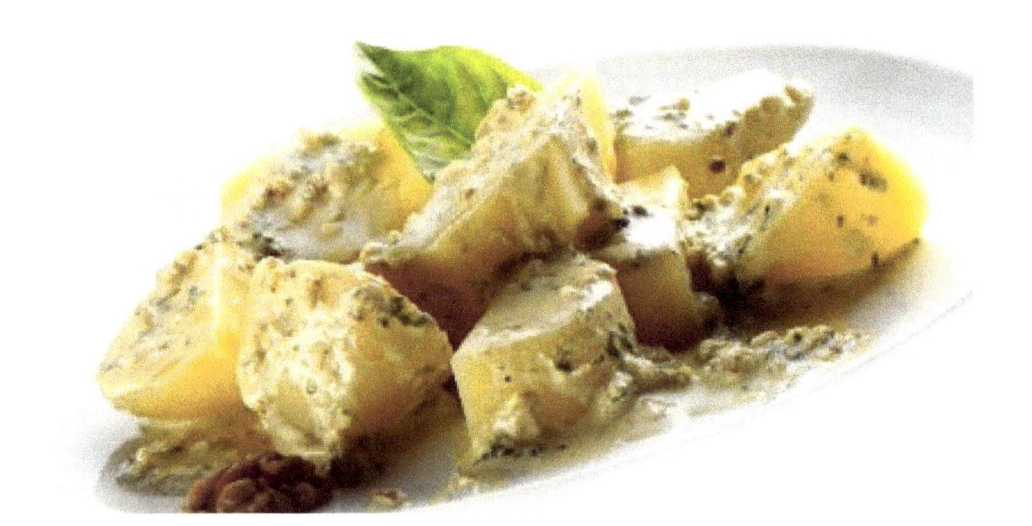

Ingredients

- 2 reddish potatoes
- 4 cups of cold water, to soak the potatoes
- 1 tsp of vegetable oil
- ½ tsp garlic powder
- 1/3 tsp of paprika
- 2 oz. feta cheese
- 1 tsp parsley, chopped
- ½ tsp of fresh oregano
- Salt and pepper
- Lemon wedges, to serve

Steps to Cook

1. Cut the potatoes into 76 x 13 mm strips and soak them in water for 15 minutes.

2. Drain the potatoes, rinse them in cold water, and dry them with paper towels. Add oil, garlic powder, and paprika to the potatoes until well covered.

3. Select Preheat, in the air fryer adjust the temperature to 195°C. Add the potatoes to the preheated air fryer.

4. Select French Fries, set the time to 28 minutes. Make sure to shake the baskets to ensure even cooking.

5. Remove the baskets from the air fryer when done cooking and cover the potatoes with feta cheese, parsley, oregano, salt and pepper. Serve with lemon wedges.

Nutritional Information

- Calories: 316
- Carbohydrates: 58.5g
- Fat: 6.9g
- Protein: 6.3g
- Sugar: 4.2g
- Cholesterol: 0mg

Omelette With Ham And Cheese

• Servings: 4 • Preparation time: 5 minutes • Cook time: 15 minutes •

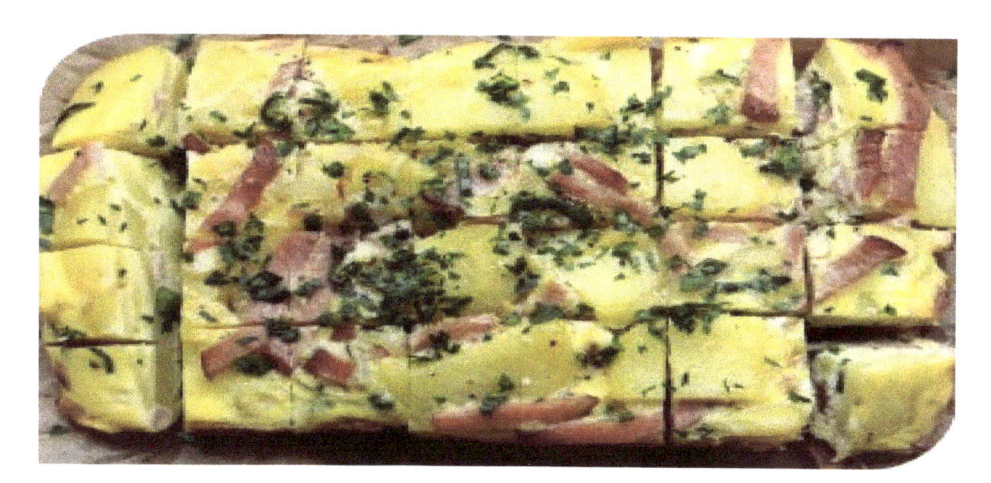

FLAVORFUL

Ingredients

- 2 large potatoes
- 5 eggs
- 1 green onion
- 1 tbsp of chopped parsley
- ½ red pepper
- 3 ½ oz. of cured ham
- 3 ½ oz. of Président Semi-cured Cheese
- 1 tbsp of olive oil
- Salt

Steps to Cook

1. Peel and cut the potatoes into thin slices. Drizzle the potatoes with a little oil.

2. Preheat the Air fryer for a few minutes at 200ºC.

3. Then place the potatoes in the basket of the Air fryer and set the timer for 10 minutes at 200ºC. Reserve.

4. Then cut the onion, pepper and parsley. In a bowl beat the eggs, add the cream cheese and season with salt and pepper to taste. Mix the beaten eggs with the potatoes, the vegetables and the diced ham.

5. Preheat the Air fryer for about 3 minutes at 180ºC.

6. While passing the mixture in a mold and putting it in the basket of the Air fryer.

7. Set the timer about 10 minutes at 180ºC temperature.

8. Turn the omelette over. Let the omelette rest for about 10 minutes inside the Air fryer

Nutritional Information

- Calories: 363
- Carbohydrates: 22g
- Fat: 19g
- Protein: 26g
- Sugar: 5g
- Cholesterol: 295mg

Chicken Skewers

• Servings: 2-4 • Preparation time: 5 minutes • Cook time: 15 minutes •

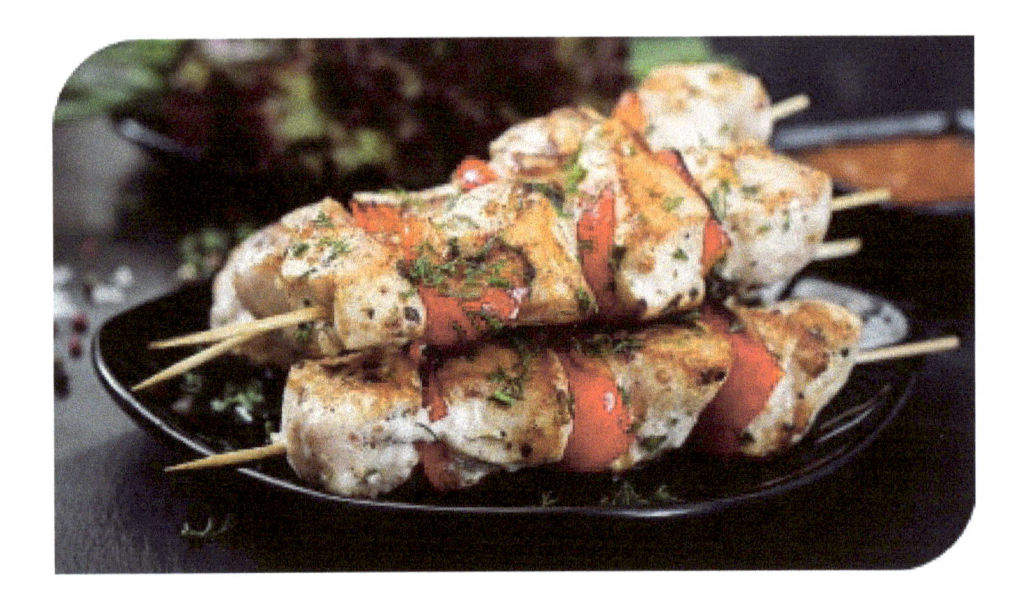

DELICIOUS
―――

Ingredients

- ½ lb boneless, skinless chicken breast
- 1 tbsp mustard
- ¼ tsp paprika
- white onion to taste
- Fine herbs
- Salt and pepper
- Wooden skewer sticks

Steps to Cook

1. Cut the chicken into large cubes and add the mustard, salt, pepper and fine herbs
2. Cut the onion and paprika into squares
3. Assemble the skewers and put them in the Air Fryer at 360°C for about 15 minutes.

Nutritional Information

- Calories: 130
- Carbohydrates: 3g
- Fat: 2.5g
- Protein: 23g
- Sugar: 4g
- Cholesterol: 65mg

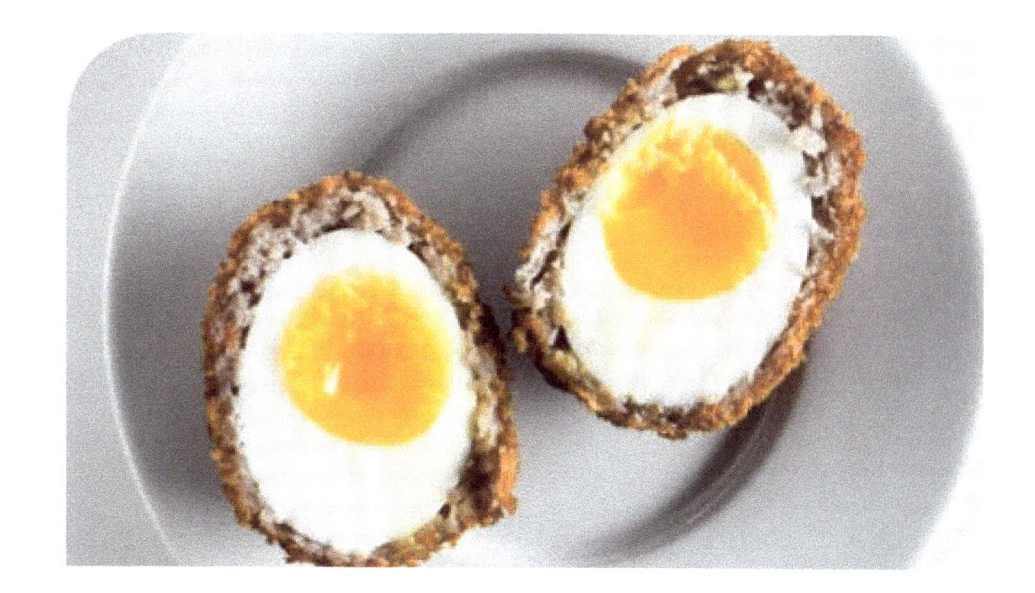

FRIED EGG

Scottish Style Egg

• Servings: 4 • Preparation time: 10 minutes • Cook time: 15 minutes •

Ingredients

- 1 lb ground pork sausage
- ¼ tsp garlic powder
- 1/3 tsp of onion powder
- 1/3 tsp of dried sage
- ¼ tsp of salt
- 1/3 tsp black pepper
- 4 eggs, half boiled, peeled
- 2 oz. all purpose flour
- 1 egg, beaten
- 1 ½ oz. Italian-style breadcrumbs Non-stick cooking spray

Steps to Cook

1. Mix together the sausage, garlic powder, onion powder, sage, salt, and pepper. Divide into four balls.

2. Wrap the sausage around each of the half-peeled hard-boiled eggs until the egg is completely covered.

3. Cover each sausage-covered egg with flour, then dip them in beaten egg and roll over breadcrumbs. Dip them again in beaten egg and pass them one last time over breadcrumbs.

4. Select Preheat, set the temperature to 175°C and Spray the eggs liberally with cooking spray.

5. Place the Scottish eggs in the preheated air fryer. Set the time to 15 minutes.

Nutritional Information

- Calories: 188
- Carbohydrates: 16g
- Fat: 6g
- Protein: 12g
- Sugar: 2g
- Cholesterol: 300mg

Avocado Burger

• Servings: 8 • Preparation time: 5 minutes • Cook time: 55 minutes •

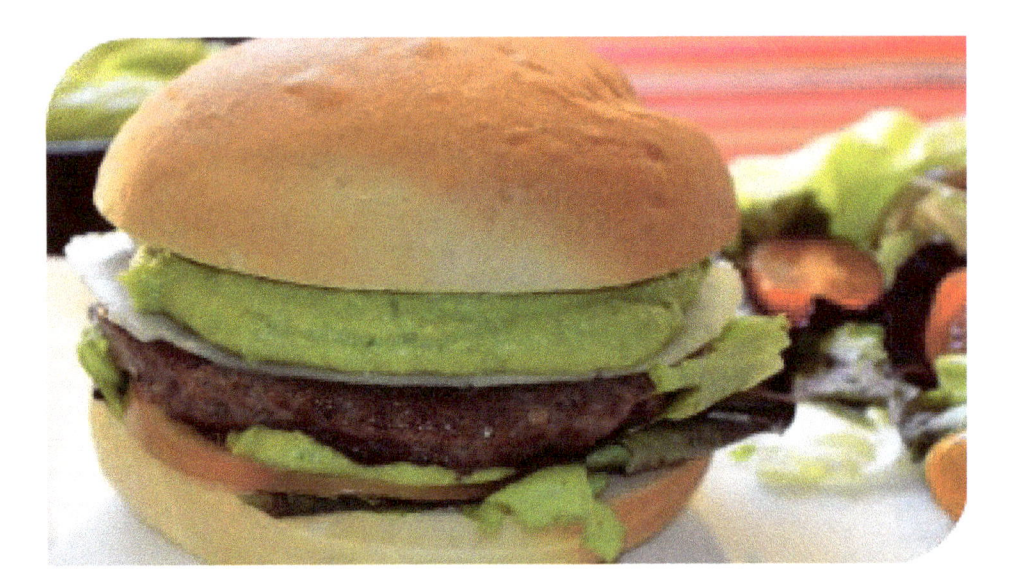

MOUTH WATERING

Ingredients

- 2 hamburger buns
- 1 lb low fat ground beef
- Red bell pepper to taste
- White onion to taste
- 2 garlic cloves
- Salt and pepper
- 2 slices of cheese
- ¼ cup ripe avocado
- 2 lettuce leaves
- 4 tomato slices

Steps to Cook

1. Blend the onion, paprika, garlic and mix it with the meat.

2. Add salt and pepper.

3. Assemble the hamburger meats and put in the Air Fryer at 360ºC for approximately 10 minutes.

4. When the meat is ready, assemble the hamburgers with tomato, cheese, lettuce and avocado slices.

Nutritional Information

- Calories: 810
- Carbohydrates: 53g
- Fat: 51g
- Protein: 36g
- Sugar: 7g
- Cholesterol: 85mg

5-Ingredient Vegetables

• Servings: 2 • Preparation time: 1h • Cook time: 30 minutes •

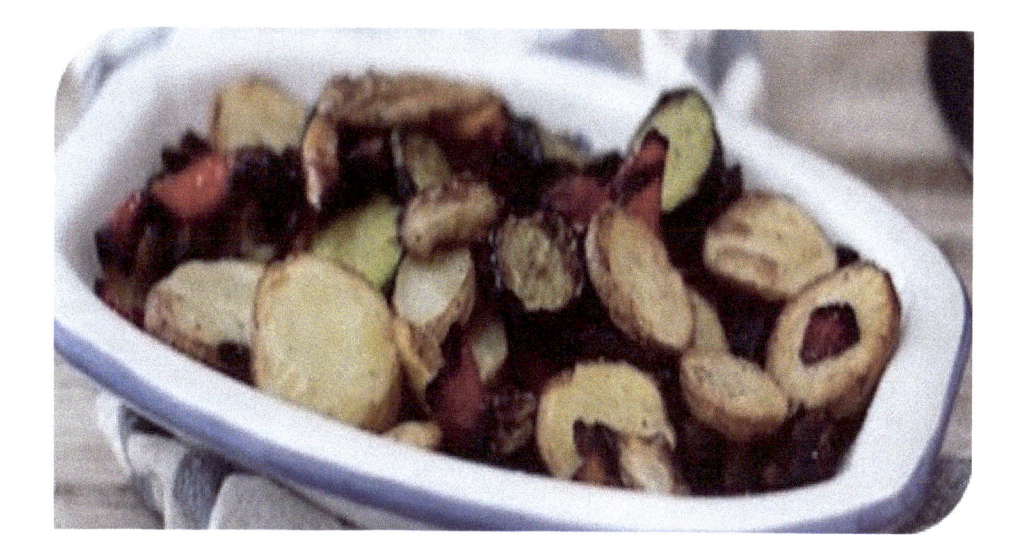

HEALTHY

Ingredients

- 2 potatoes
- 1 zucchini
- 1 onion
- 1 red pepper
- 1 green pepper

Steps to Cook

1. Cut the potatoes into slices.

2. Cut the onion into rings

3. Cut the zucchini slices

4. Cut the peppers into strips.

5. Put all in one bowl and add a little salt, ground pepper and a few strands of extra virgin olive oil.

6. Mix well.

7. Go to the basket of the Air fryer.

8. Select 160ºC for 30 minutes.

9. Check that the vegetables are to our liking.

Nutritional Information

- Calories: 117.6
- Carbohydrates: 13.4g
- Fat: 6.9g
- Protein: 1.8g
- Sugar: 4g
- Cholesterol: 0mg

Loin Rolls

• Servings: 12 • Preparation time: 10 minutes • Cook time: 40 minutes •

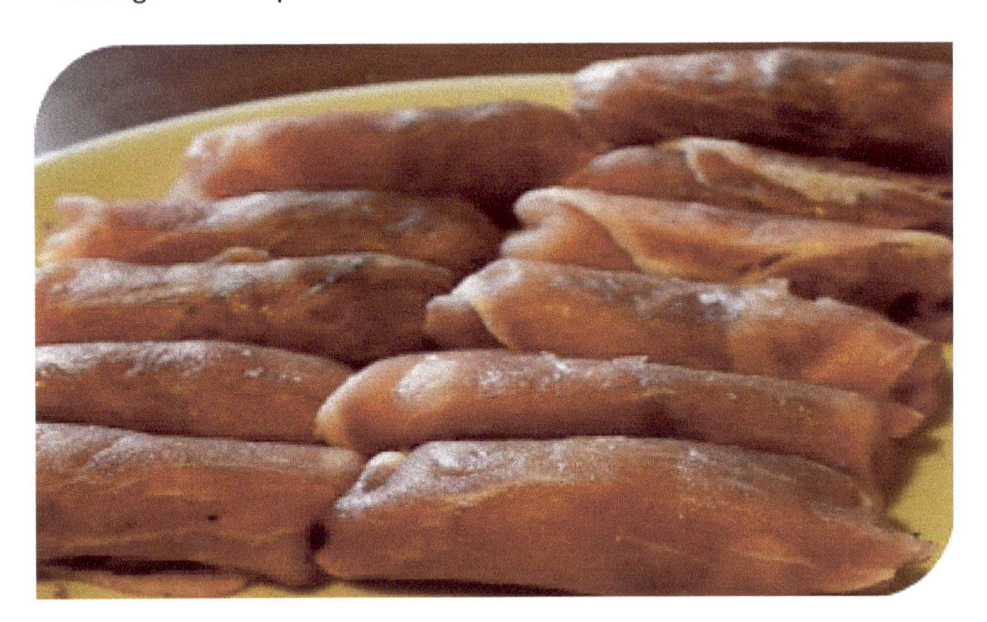

DELICIOUS

Ingredients

- 12 tenderloin steaks
- 12 strips of soft cheese
- 6 slices of bacon
- Extra virgin olive oil
- Salt
- Ground pepper

Steps to Cook

1. Add salt and pepper to the fillets and spread on the worktable.

2. Place on each fillet a slice of bacon and a strip of soft cheese.

3. Roll up.

4. Place on a tray suitable for the air fryer.

5. Season with salt and pepper and add a few strands of extra virgin olive oil.

6. Take to the air fryer, 170ºC about 40 minutes.

Nutritional Information

- Calories: 55.3
- Carbohydrates: 0g
- Fat: 2.2g
- Protein: 8.4g
- Sugar: 0g
- Cholesterol: 22.1mg

Grilled Fillet Steaks

• Servings: 4 • Preparation time 5 minutes • Cook time: 20-25 minutes •

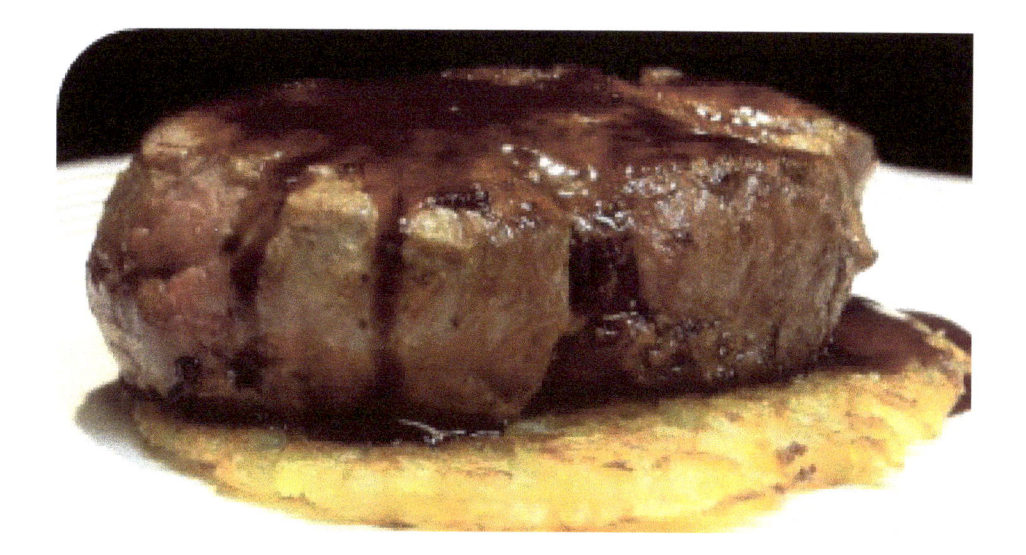

YUMMY

Ingredients

- 8 tenderloin steaks
- ½ lb of kale
- 4 cloves of garlic
- Extra virgin olive oil
- Salt
- Ground pepper
- Grated cheese

Steps to Cook

1. Put in the Wok a base of extra virgin olive oil with the rolled garlic. When the garlic begins to sauté, add the chopped kale and sauté until you see it at its point. Season with salt and pepper and transfer to a tray suitable for the air fryer.

2. In a frying pan with a little oil, make the fillets of loin previously seasoned. Pass them on both sides and place on the sauteed Kale.

3. Cover everything with a layer of grated cheese.

4. Take to the air fryer, 180ºC, until the cheese melts, about 20-25 minutes.

Nutritional Information

- Calories: 179
- Carbohydrates: 0g
- Fat: 7.6g
- Protein: 26g
- Sugar: 0g
- Cholesterol: 79mg

Chapter 4

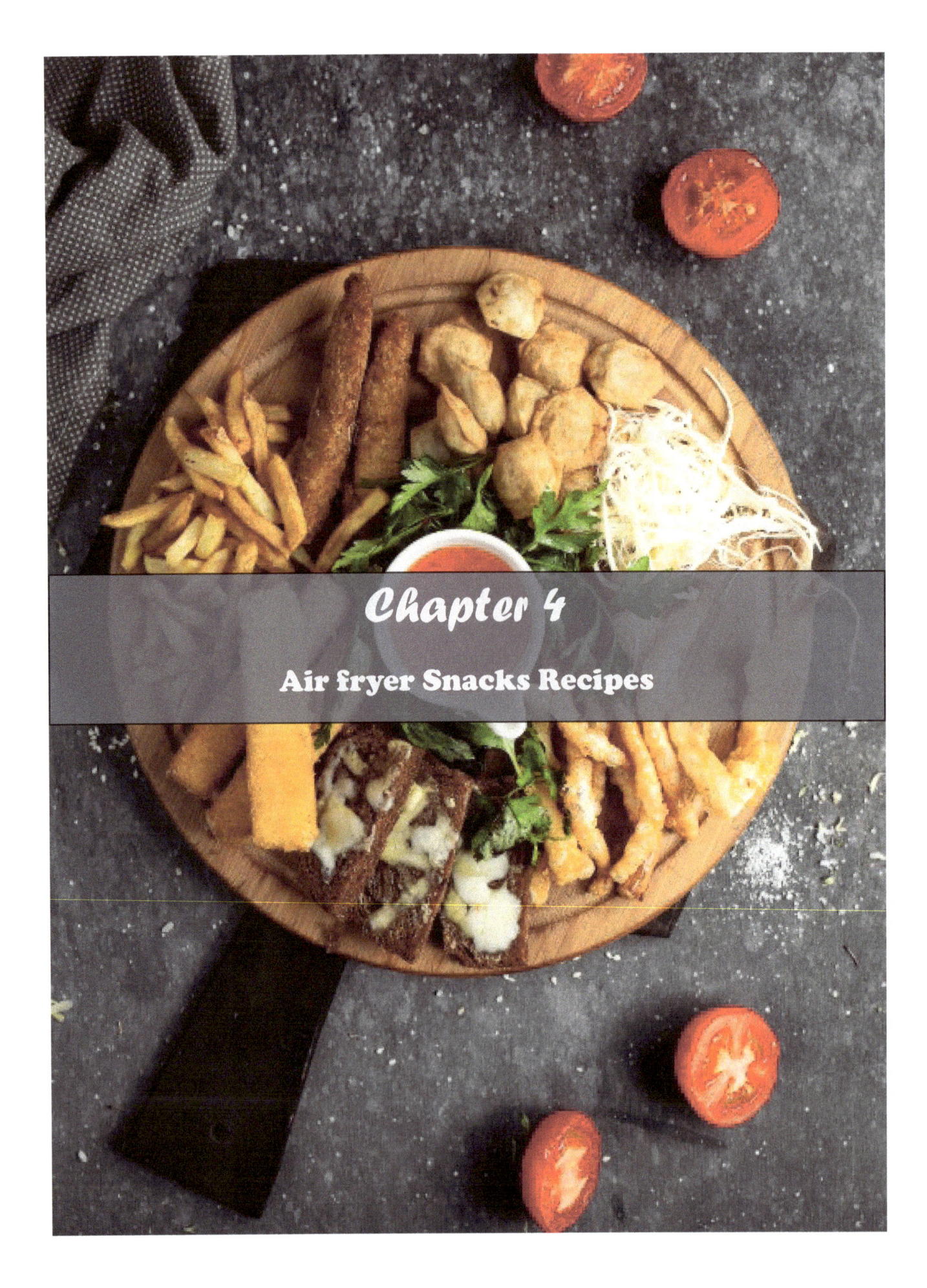

Air fryer Snacks Recipes

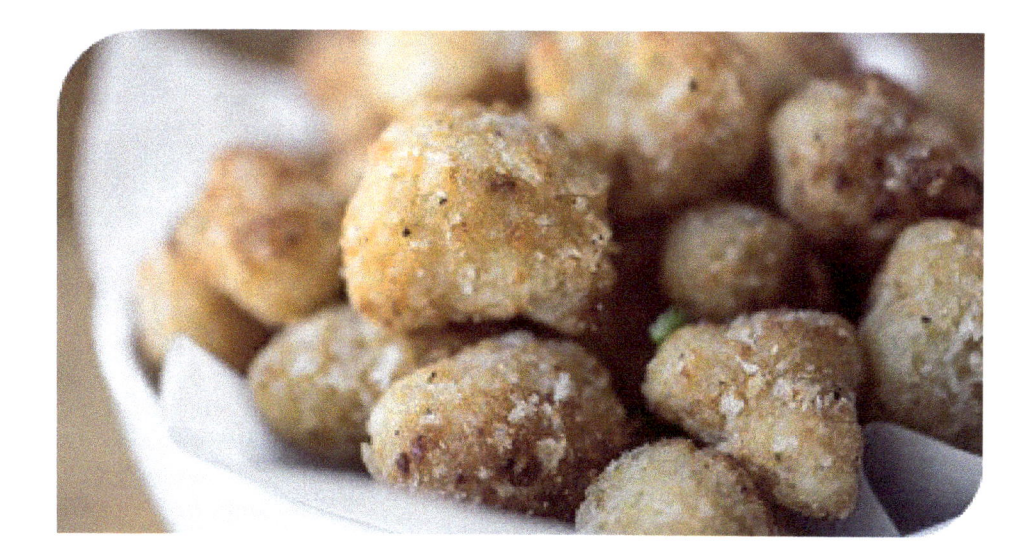

QUICK & EASY

Cauliflower Pops

• Servings: 2 • Preparation time: 5 minutes • Cook time: 15 minutes •

Ingredients

- Kitchen spray
- 4 cup cauliflower
- 1 large egg,
- 1 cup Shredded cheddar
- 1 cup grated parmesan
- 2/3 cup panko bread-crumbs
- 2 tbsp freshly chives.
- Kosher salt
- Freshly ground black pepper
- ½ cup ketchup
- 2 tbsp Sriracha

Steps to Cook

1. Cook the cauliflower until just done. Place the cooked cauliflower on a clean kitchen towel and squeeze to drain the water. In a food processor, grind the cauliflower with the intention of making it similar to rice. Transfer the cauliflower to a large bowl with egg, cheddar, parmesan, panko, and chives, and mix until combined. Season with salt and pepper to taste.

2. With a spoon, take the mixture and roll it into a potato shape. Working in batches, arrange them in a single layer air fryer basket and cook at 375° for 10 minutes. Meanwhile, make spicy ketchup: Combine ketchup and Sriracha in a small bowl and stir to combine.

3. Serve hot cauliflower pops with spicy ketchup.

Nutritional Information

- Calories: 51.4
- Carbohydrates: 3.2g
- Fat: 2.9g
- Protein: 3.3g
- Sugar: 0.5g
- Cholesterol: 9.3mg

Air Fryer Cookbook

Onion Rings

• Servings: 2 • Preparation time: 1 minutes • Cook time: 20 minutes •

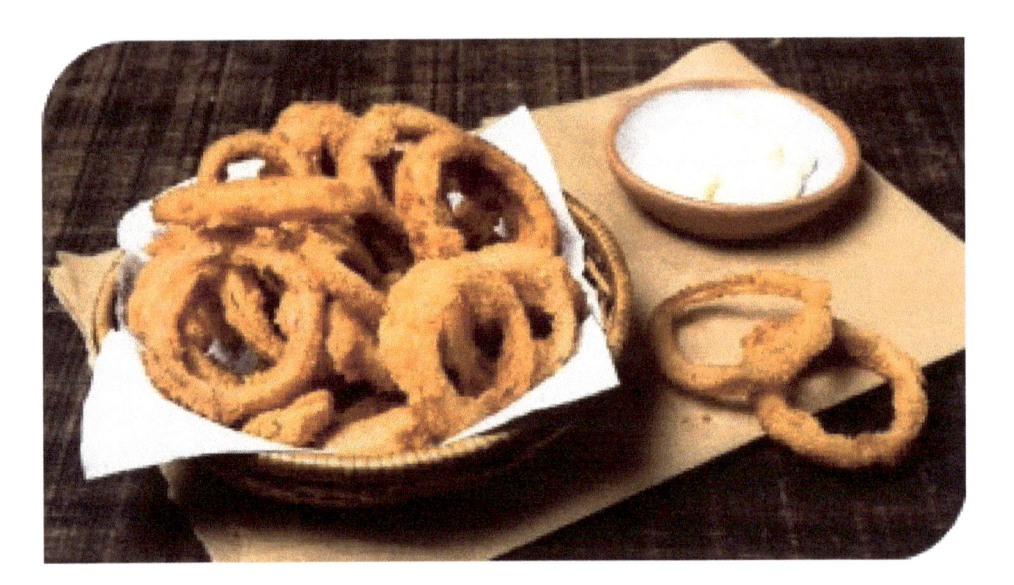

CRUNCHY

Ingredients

- 1 small white onion, cut into 13mm thick rounds and separated into rings
- 3 oz. of crusty breadcrumbs
- 1/3 tsp smoked paprika
- 1 tsp of salt
- 2 eggs
- 1 cup whey
- 2 oz. all-purpose flour
- Non-stick spray oil

Steps to Cook

1. Cut an onion into 13mm thick slices and separate the layers into rings.

2. Combine the breadcrumbs, paprika, and salt in a bowl. Leave aside.

3. Beat the eggs and buttermilk until completely mixed.

4. Dip each onion ring into the flour, then into the beaten eggs, and finally into the breadcrumb mixture.

5. Select Preheat on the air fryer, set it to 190°C.

6. Pour the onion rings liberally with cooking oil.

7. Arrange the onion rings in a single layer in the baskets of the preheated air fryer and cook in batches at 190 ° C for 10 minutes until golden. Make sure to use cooking spray halfway through cooking so they cook evenly.

8. Serve with your favorite sauce.

Nutritional Information

- Calories: 304
- Carbohydrates: 31g
- Fat: 18g
- Protein: 3.8g
- Sugar: 1g
- Cholesterol: 1mg

Feta Cheese in the Shape of Triangles

• Servings: 4-6 • Preparation time: 5 minutes • Cook time: 3 minutes •

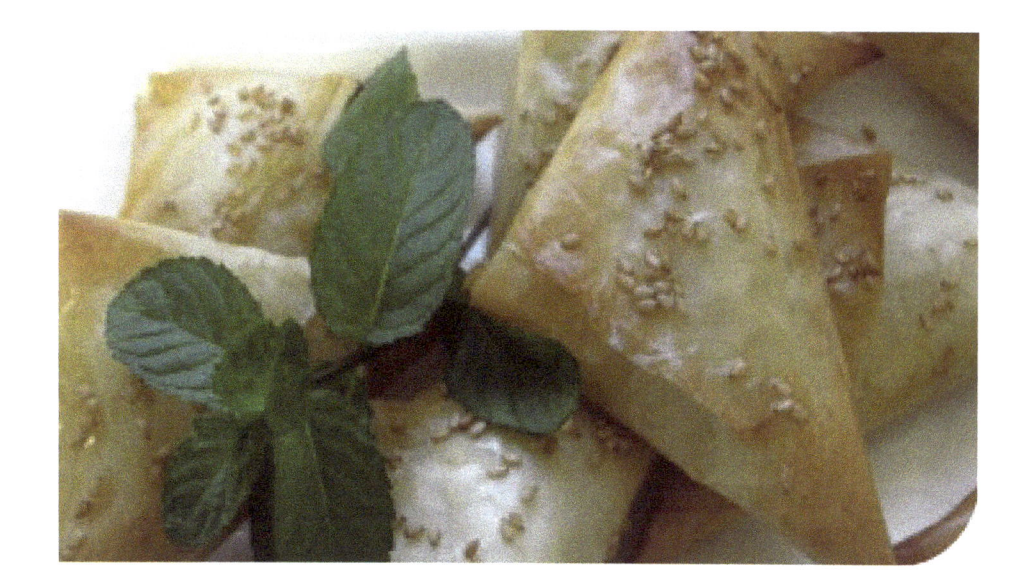

RICH COLESTEROL

Ingredients

- 1 egg yolk
- 3 ½ oz. of feta cheese
- 2 tbsp of chopped parsley
- 1 chive in fine rings
- Freshly ground black pepper
- 5 sheets of frozen phyllo dough

Steps to Cook

1. Beat the egg yolk in a bowl and mix it with the feta cheese, parsley and chives; season with pepper to taste.

2. Cut each sheet of phyllo into three strips.

3. Take a full teaspoon of the feta mixture and place it on the inside of a strip of pasta.

4. Fold the point of the pasta over the filling to form a triangle, and then fold the point in zigzag until the filling is wrapped in a triangle of pasta.

5. Fill the other strips of pasta with feta in the same way. Preheat the air fryer to 200°C. Brush the triangles with a little oil and put five of them in the basket. Insert the basket into the air fryer and set the timer to 3 minutes.

Nutritional Information

- Calories: 89
- Carbohydrates: 11.7g
- Fat: 3.6g
- Protein: 3g
- Sugar: 0.3g
- Cholesterol: 300mg

Air Fryer Cookbook

Meat and cheese patty

Ingredients

• Servings: 4 • Preparation time: 5 minutes • Cook time: 15 minutes •

For the mass:
- 3 c. all-purpose flour plus more for the surface
- 1 teaspoon of kosher salt
- 1 tsp baking powder
- ½ cup cold butter, diced
- ¾ cup of water
- 1 large egg

For the filling:
- 1 tbsp of extra virgin olive oil
- 1 yellow onion, chopped
- 2 garlic cloves, minced
- 1 pound ground beef
- 1 tbsp of tomato paste
- 1 tsp of oregano
- 1 tsp of cumin
- ½ tsp of paprika
- Kosher salt
- Freshly ground black pepper
- ½ cup chopped tomatoes
- ½ cup chopped pickled jalapeños
- 1 ¼ cup grated cheddar
- 1 ¼ cup Monterey Jack crushed
- Egg washing, for brushing
- Freshly chopped coriander, for garnish
- Sour cream, to serve

Steps to Cook

1. In a large skillet over medium heat, heat the oil. Add onion and cook until smooth, about 5 minutes, then add garlic and cook until fragrant, 1 more minute.

2. Add the ground meat and cook, breaking the meat with a wooden spoon, until it is no longer pink, 5 minutes. Drain the fat.

3. Put the skillet back on medium heat and stir the tomato paste into the meat. Add the oregano, cumin and paprika and season with salt and pepper.

4. Add the tomatoes and jalapeños and cook until heated through, about 3 minutes. Remove from heat and allow to cool slightly.

5. Place the dough on a lightly floured surface and divide it in half. Roll one half until it is ¼ "thick. Using a 4.5 " round cookie cutter, cut off the roundings. Repeat with the rest of the dough.

6. Rewind the pieces once to cut more rounds.

7. Lightly moisten the outer edge of a round of dough with water and place about 2 tablespoons of filling in the center and cover with cheddar and Monterey.

8. Fold the dough in half over the filling.

9. Use a fork to join the edges, and then brush with washed egg.

10. Repeat with the rest of the filling and the dough.

11. Place the empanadas in a parchment-lined compressed air basket, making sure they don't touch, and cook them in batches at 400° for 10 minutes.

12. Garnish with coriander and serve with sour cream.

Nutritional Information

- Calories: 350
- Carbohydrates: 36g
- Fat: 14g
- Protein: 12g
- Sugar: 5g
- Cholesterol: 275mg

Grilled Pineapple

• Servings: 4 • Preparation time: 10 minutes • Cook time: 15 minutes •

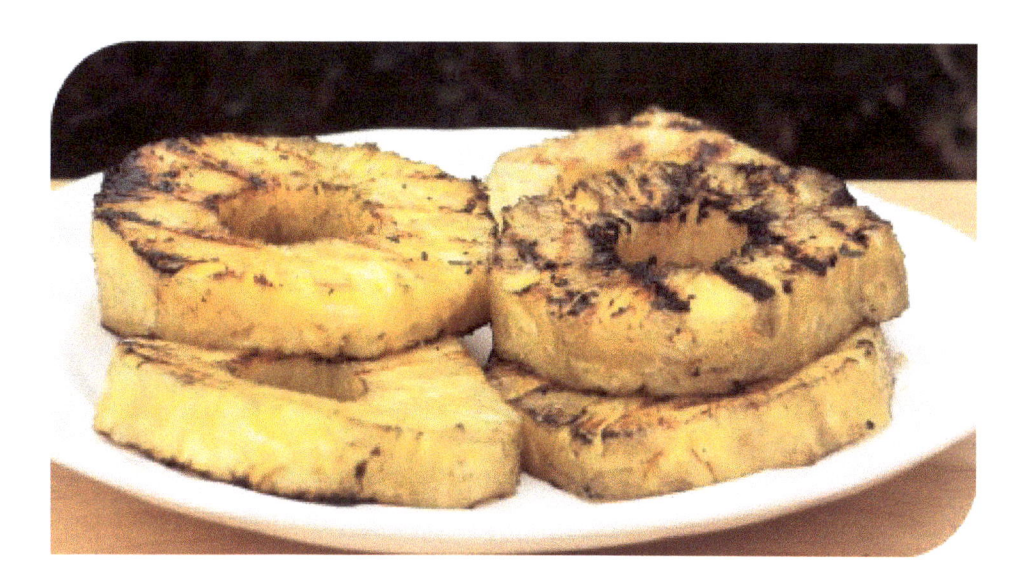

FRUITY

Ingredients

- 8 pineapple slices in their juice
- Lemon yogurt
- 4 chopped walnuts
- Strawberry and/or honey syrup

Steps to Cook

1. Open a small can of pineapple, drain well.

2. Preheat the Air fryer to a temperature of 200ºC.

3. Place the pineapple slices in the basket of the Air fryer.

4. Set the Air fryer's timer for about 10 minutes at 200°C, at medium cooking turn each slice and end the cooking time.

5. Serve the roasted pineapple on each plate, with lemon yogurt or vanilla ice cream.

6. Add the chopped walnuts on top and sauce with syrup strawberries or honey.

Nutritional Information

- Calories: 67.1
- Carbohydrates: 17.1g
- Fat: 0.4g
- Protein: 0.3g
- Sugar: 0g
- Cholesterol: 0mg

Air Fryer Cookbook

Ham Triangles

• Servings: 4 • Preparation time: 5 minutes • Cook time: 10 minutes •

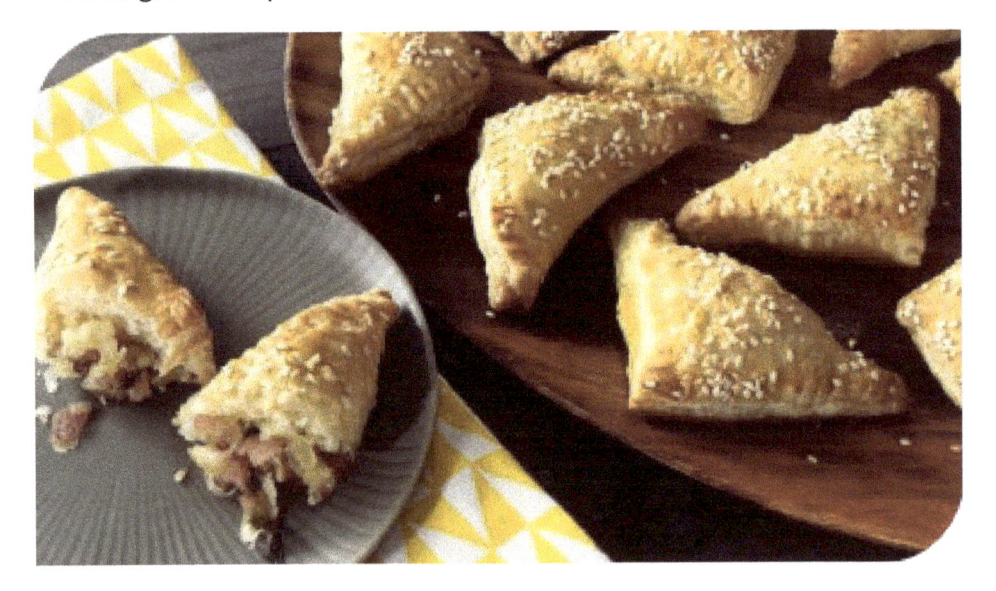

FLAVORFUL

Ingredients

- 8 slices of cooked ham
- 1 goat roll
- Egg
- Bread crumbs
- Extra virgin olive oil

Steps to Cook

1. Put the goat cheese in a bowl and squeeze well with a fork. We can also crumble with our fingers or we can chop with a knife. Spread the slices of cooked ham well on the work table.

2. Distribute the goat roll between the 8 slices, placing a ball in each corner of the slice of cooked ham.

3. Wrap the goat roll with the cooked ham so that we have some triangles.

4. Take to the freezer 30 minutes.

5. Go through beaten egg, through breadcrumbs, again through beaten egg and finish with breadcrumbs.

6. Leave in the freezer 15 minutes.

7. Put in the air fryer at 200ºC for 10 minutes.

Nutritional Information

- Calories: 89
- Carbohydrates: 11.7g
- Fat: 3.6g
- Protein: 3g
- Sugar: 0.3g
- Cholesterol: 300mg

Mini Apple-Flavored Empanadas

• Servings: 2 • Preparation time: 35 minutes • Cook time: 10 minutes •

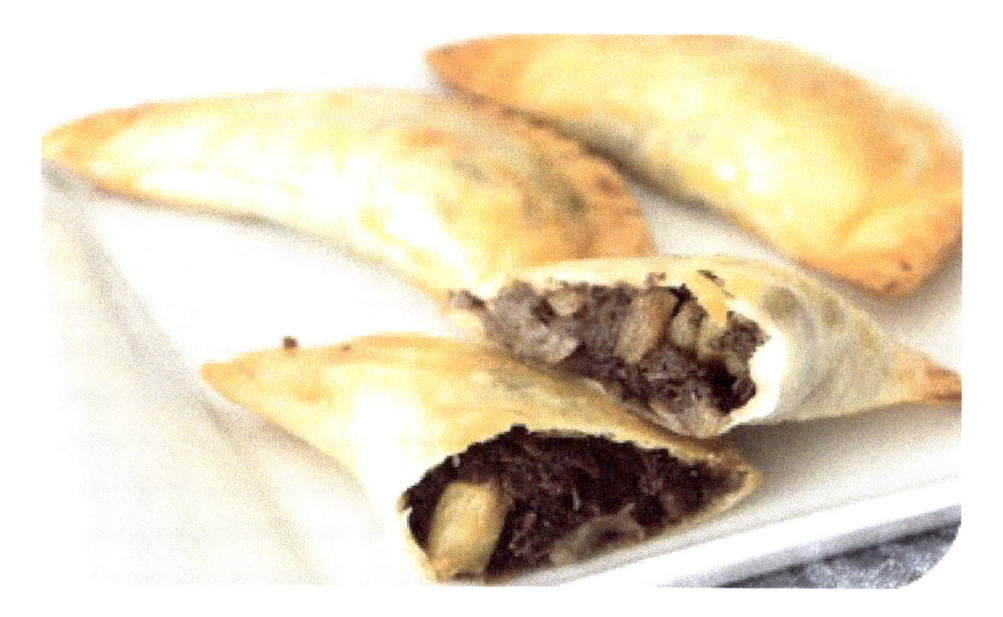

LOVELY

Ingredients

- 1 medium apple, peeled and diced
- ½ oz granulated sugar
- ½ oz. unsalted butter
- 1/3 tsp ground cinnamon
- ¼ tsp of ground nutmeg
- ¼ tsp of ground allspice
- 1 sheet of pre-made cake batter
- 1 beaten egg
- 1 tsp milk

Steps to Cook

1. Combine diced apples, granulated sugar, butter, cinnamon, nutmeg, and allspice in a medium saucepan or skillet over medium-low heat.

2. Simmer for 2 minutes and remove from heat.

3. Cut the cake batter into 127mm circles.

4. Add the filling to the center of each circle and use your finger to apply water to the outer ends. Some filler will be left unused.

5. Close the cake by cutting a small opening at the top.

6. Select Preheat, in the air fryer adjust the temperature to 175°C.

7. Mix the eggs and milk and roll the mixture over each foot. Place the cakes in the preheated air fryer and cook at 175°C for 10 minutes until the cakes are browned.

Nutritional Information

- Calories: 154
- Carbohydrates: 11.94g
- Fat: 12.05g
- Protein: 1.69g
- Sugar: 5.22g
- Cholesterol: 0mg

Air Fryer Cookbook

Homemade Churros

• Servings: 2-4 • Preparation time: 15 minutes• Cook time: 1-5 minutes •

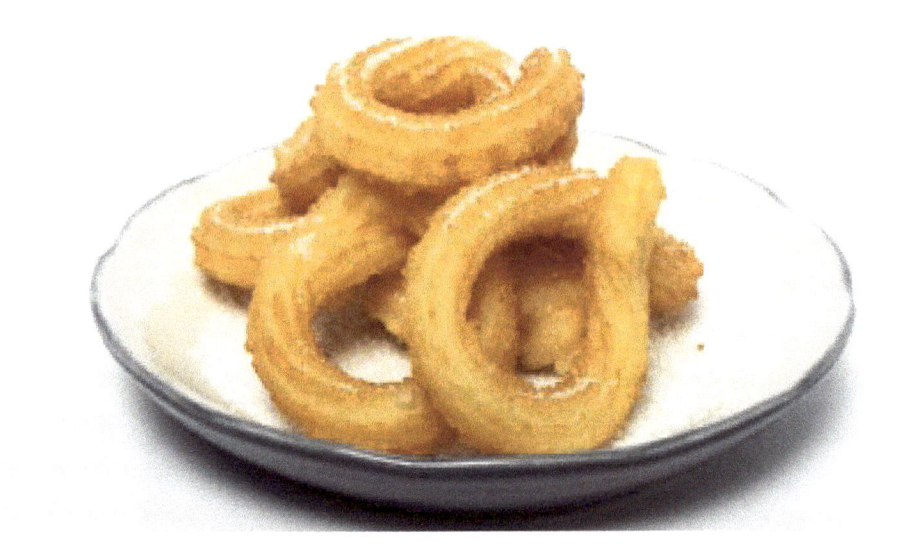

VERY QUICK

Ingredients

- 1 cup of water
- 1 cup plain all-purpose flour
- 1 tsp salt
- A churros machine

Steps to Cook

1. In a saucepan, add the water and salt until it starts to boil. Suddenly add the flour and with a wooden spoon start stirring quickly until there is no more liquid.

2. Dump the dough on the work table while it is hot and knead with your hands quickly, if you let it cool down this dough will become very hard and they will no longer come out ... Put in the churros machine while the dough is still hot. Go forming the churros in the form of a loop or the shape that you like the most.

3. Put in the deep air fryer at temperature of about 180ºC for 1 minute.

4. Introduce the churros separately and cover, after 1 minute turn. After 30 more seconds or when they are already golden.

Nutritional Information

- Calories: 103
- Carbohydrates: 8.4g
- Fat: 7.7g
- Protein: 0.5g
- Sugar: 4.8g
- Cholesterol: 0mg

Chips

• Servings: 4 • Preparation time: 5 minutes • Cook time: 15 minutes •

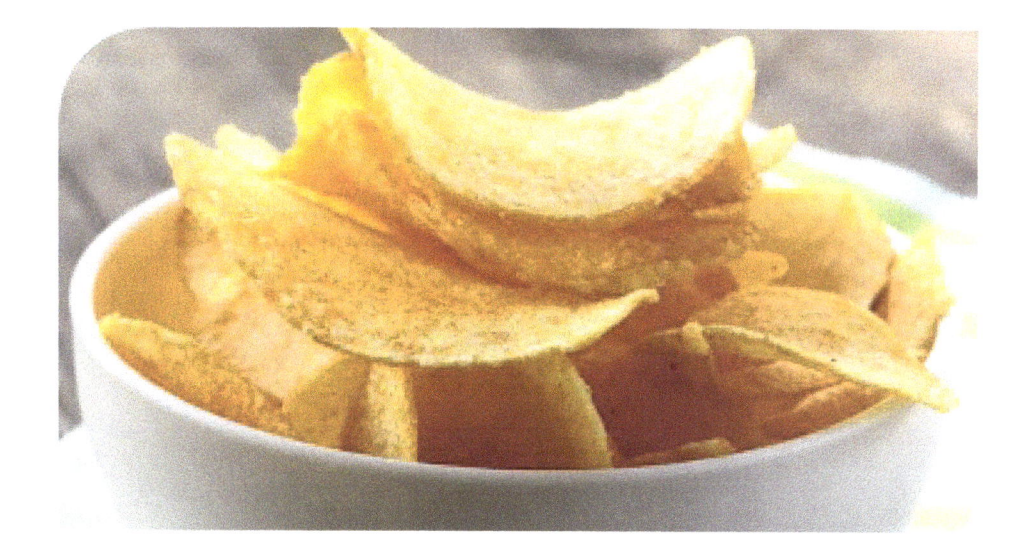

CRUNCHY

Ingredients

- The amount of potatoes you want.
- 1 tbsp of oil
- Salt.
- Special to taste

Steps to Cook

1. Peel and chop each potato. Put them in a bowl with water for 20 minutes. This will cleanse and hydrate them for a better result. Drain and pat dry a bit so they aren't dripping. Just dry them in the fryer for 10 minutes at 80ºC. Thus, they will also begin to cook so that they are made uniformly during the final cooking.

2. Add a tablespoon of oil to the potatoes so they don't stick and taste.

3. Season them to taste.

4. Now it is time to cook them in the deep fryer without oil for 30 minutes at 180ºC.

5. Stir them from time to time if your fryer doesn't have an automatic movement system.

6. It only remains to enjoy this delicious recipe.

Nutritional Information

- Calories: 152
- Carbohydrates: 15g
- Fat: 9.8g
- Protein: 2g
- Sugar: 0.1g
- Cholesterol: 75mg

Strawberry And Cream Buns

• Servings: 6 • Preparation time: 10 minutes • Cook time: 12 minutes •

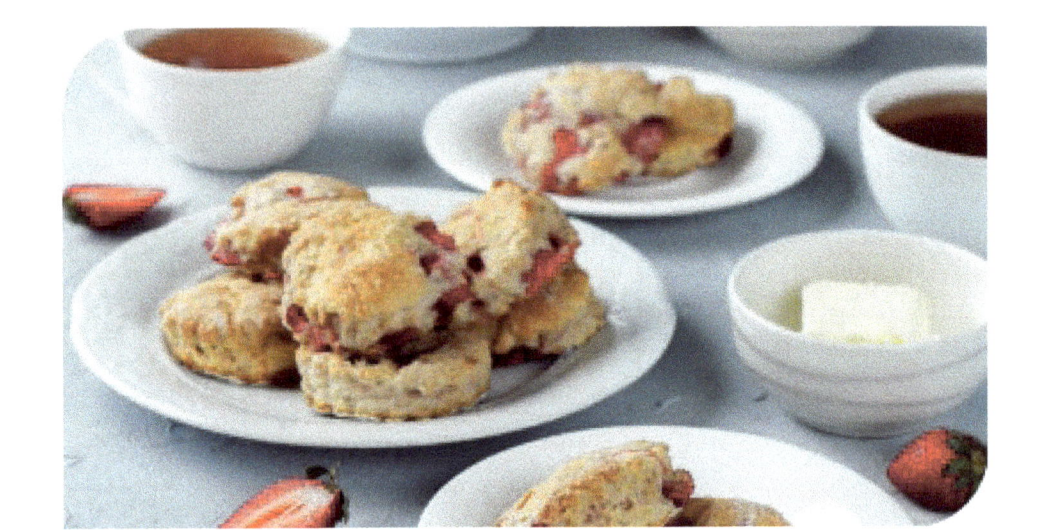

STRAWBERRY FLAVORED

Ingredients

- 9 oz. all-purpose flour
- 1.7 oz. of granulated sugar.
- 0.2 oz. baking powder
- ½ tsp of salt
- 2.8 oz. butter
- 3 oz. fresh strawberries, cut into small pieces
- ½ cup thick cream
- 2 large eggs
- 2 tsp of vanilla extract
- 1 tsp of water

Steps to Cook

1. Mix flour, sugar, baking powder, and salt in large bowl. Cut the butter into the flour with a confectionery blender or with your hands until the mixture is thick and gritty.

2. Add strawberries to mix and set aside. Whisk together the heavy cream, 1 egg and the vanilla extract in a separate bowl. Incorporate the cream mixture into the flour container until completely mixed, and flatten it to 38 cm thick. Use a cookie cutter to cut the buns. Mix 1 egg with water and use this mixture to coat the buns. Reserve. Select Preheat in the air fryer, set the temperature to 175 °C and press Start/Pause. Cover the preheated inner basket with parchment paper. Place buns on parchment paper and bake for 12 minutes at 175°C.

Nutritional Information

- Calories: 222
- Carbohydrates: 39g
- Fat: 6g
- Protein: 3g
- Sugar: 22g
- Cholesterol: 53mg

Blueberries And Gingerbread

• Servings: 6 • Preparation time: 10 minutes • Cook time: 12minutes •

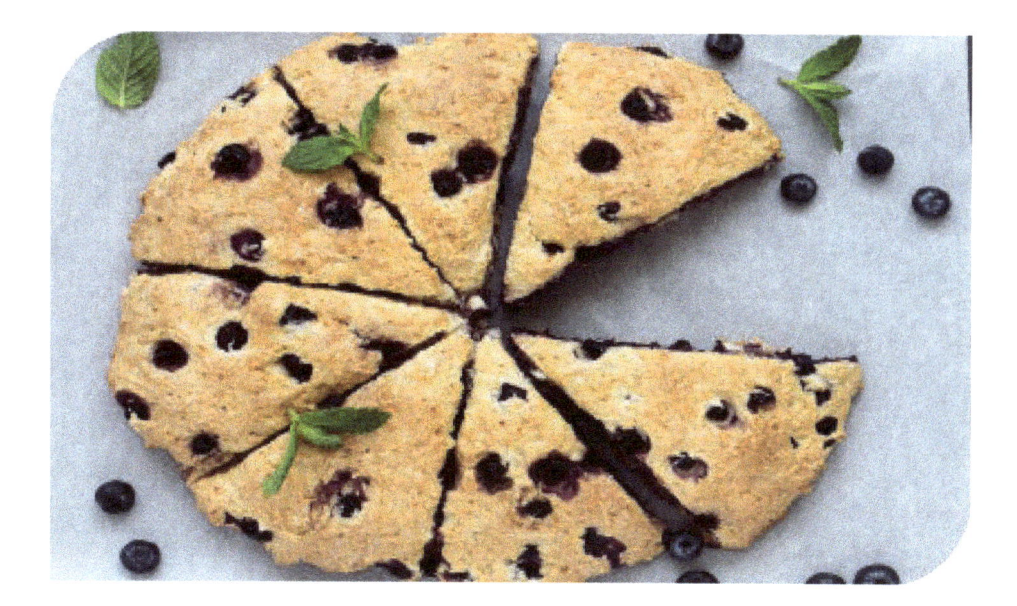

Ingredients

- 8 ½ oz. all-purpose flour
- 3 oz. granulated sugar
- 1 ½ tsp baking powder
- ½ tsp salt
- 3 oz. butter
- 3 oz. fresh blueberries
- ½ tsp finely grated fresh ginger
- ½ cup thick cream
- 2 large eggs
- 1 tsp of vanilla extract
- 1 cup of water

Steps to Cook

1. Mix flour, sugar, baking powder, and salt in large bowl. Cut the butter into the flour with a blender or with your hands until the mixture is thick.

2. Mix the blueberries and ginger with the mixture. Whisk together the heavy cream, 1 egg and the vanilla extract in a separate bowl. Add the cream mixture to the flour bowl until completely mixed. Form a round ball 38 cm thick and cut it into eighths. Mix 1 egg with water and use this mixture to coat the buns. Reserve.

3. Select Preheat, set the temperature to 175°C and press Start/Pause. Cover the preheated inner basket with parchment paper. Place buns on parchment paper and bake for 12 minutes at 175 °C.

Nutritional Information

- Calories: 266
- Carbohydrates: 41.4g
- Fat: 10g
- Protein: 3.5g
- Sugar: 24g
- Cholesterol: 16mg

Air Fryer Cookbook

Fingers of cheese with Cheetos flamin

• Servings: 4 • Preparation time: 2h 10minutes • Cook time: 5-6 minutes •

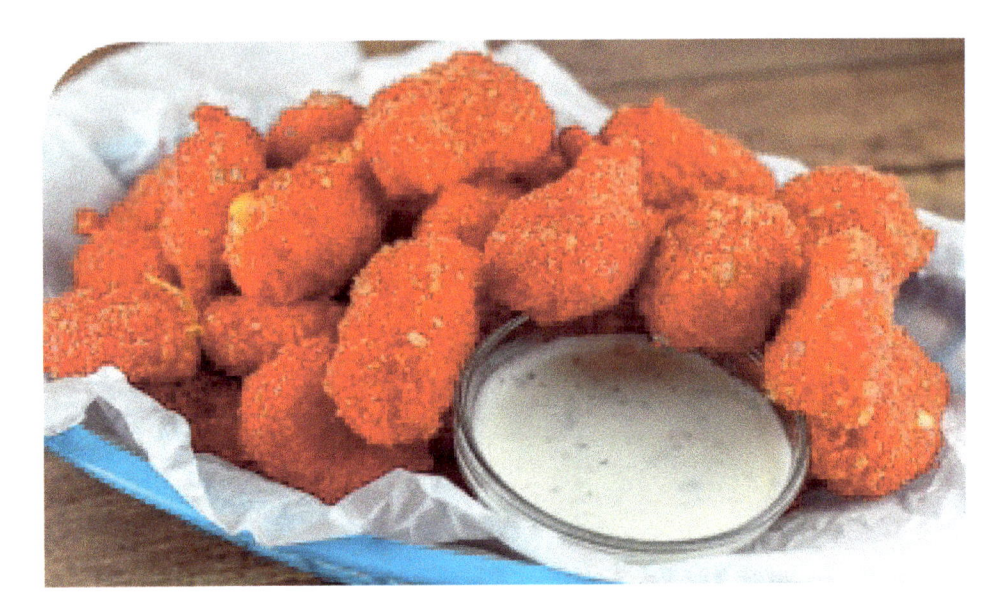

FLAVORSOME

Ingredients

- 10 mozzarella cheese sticks
- 2 eggs
- 2 cups hot Cheetos
- ½ cup flour

Steps to Cook

1. First of all put the flour on a plate, beat the eggs and put the hot Cheetos in a bag and crush them.

2. Put a cheese in the egg, then in the flour, then in the Cheetos and again in the egg and finally again in the Cheetos. Since they are all ready, put them in the freezer for about 2 hours.

3. Since they are ready, put them in the air fryer at 350°C and 3 minutes (you have to spray oil on the grate so that it does not stick). Open and turn them and put another 3 minutes, and ready.

Nutritional Information

- Calories: 73
- Carbohydrates: 12.9g
- Fat: 1.4g
- Protein: 2.5g
- Sugar: 2.7g
- Cholesterol: 13.6mg

Roasted Apples

• Servings: 4 • Preparation time: 5 minutes • Cook time: 18 minutes •

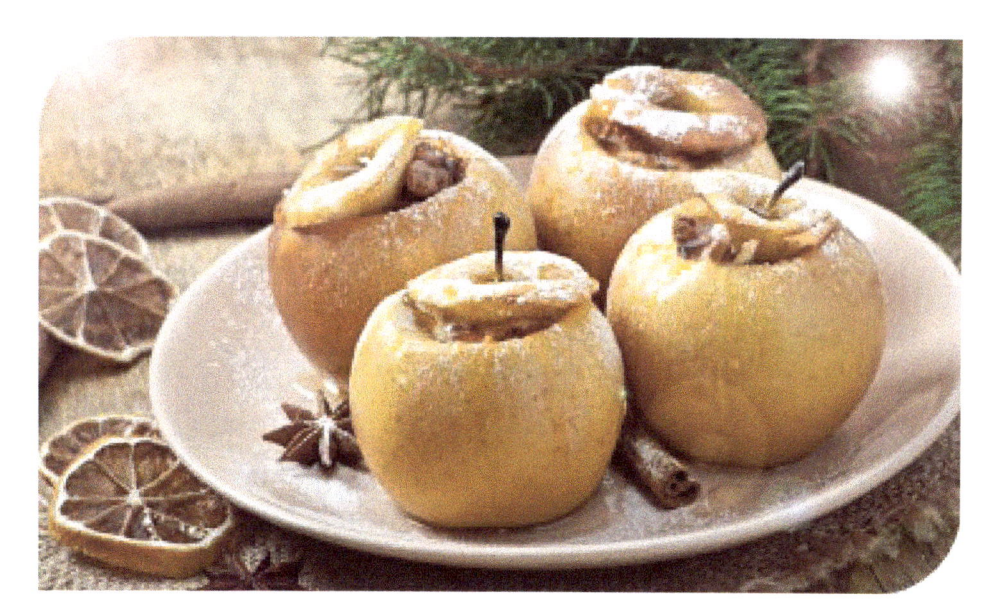

MOUTHWATERING

Ingredients

- 4 apples
- 4 teaspoons sweet milk
- ice cream to serve and mint to serve

Steps to Cook

1. Wash the apples and with a lace remove a large part of the apple pit. Put a small amount of sweet milk in the hole (you can also add sugar and a little bit of muscat). Put them in the basket and program 180°C 18 minutes when the time is up to see if they are ready and remove. If you see that it is missing a little leave them 2 more minutes.

2. Let cool and serve with a spoon of lemon ice cream and some mint leaves. A healthy, fast and deliciously rich dessert.

Nutritional Information

- Calories: 173
- Carbohydrates: 39g
- Fat: 1.9g
- Protein: 0.8g
- Sugar: 32g
- Cholesterol: 7.8mg

Grilled Razors

• Servings: 4• Preparation time: 5 minutes• Cook time: 8minutes •

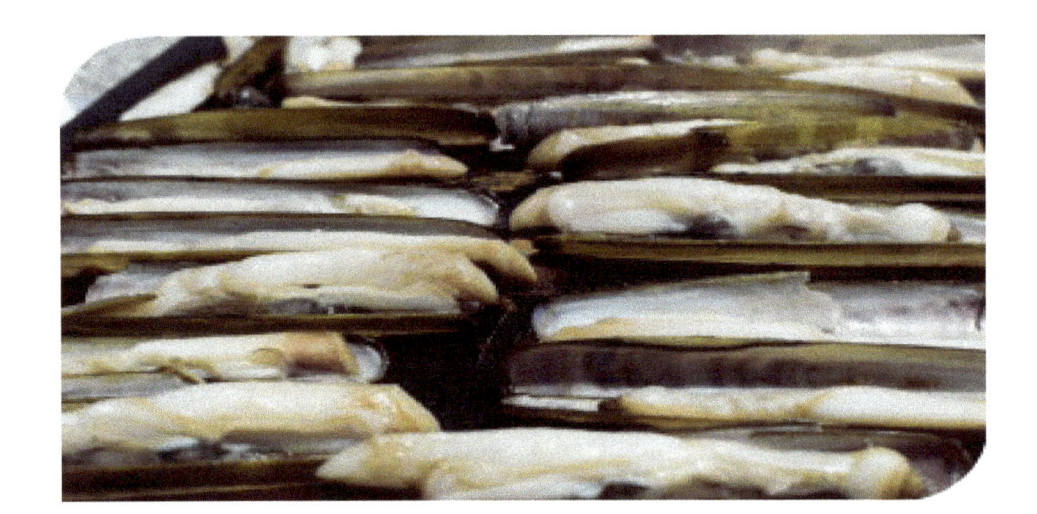

FANTASTIC

Ingredients

- 1 mesh of live razors
- The juice of a lime
- Fresh parsley, very minced
- 4 cloves garlic, very minced
- Salt
- Coarse salt to clean the razors

Steps to Cook

1. Soak the razors with coarse salt so that they release the sand. It is best to put them vertically a minimum of 20 minutes.

2. Mix the ingredients for the dressing.

3. Heat the air fryer to 240ºC for 5 minutes.

4. Clarify and drain the razors. Paint the bucket with the dressing with the help of a silicone brush. Put the razors and leave until they have a nice golden color. In 3 minutes they are open and done. Paint with the dressing a couple of times, at least, during the process.

5. When serving put salt broken between your fingers.

Nutritional Information

- Calories: 88
- Carbohydrates: 0.6g
- Fat: 1.08g
- Protein: 17.95g
- Sugar: 0g
- Cholesterol: 63mg

Marranitas

• Servings: 2-4 • Preparation time: 5 minutes • Cook time: 57minutes •

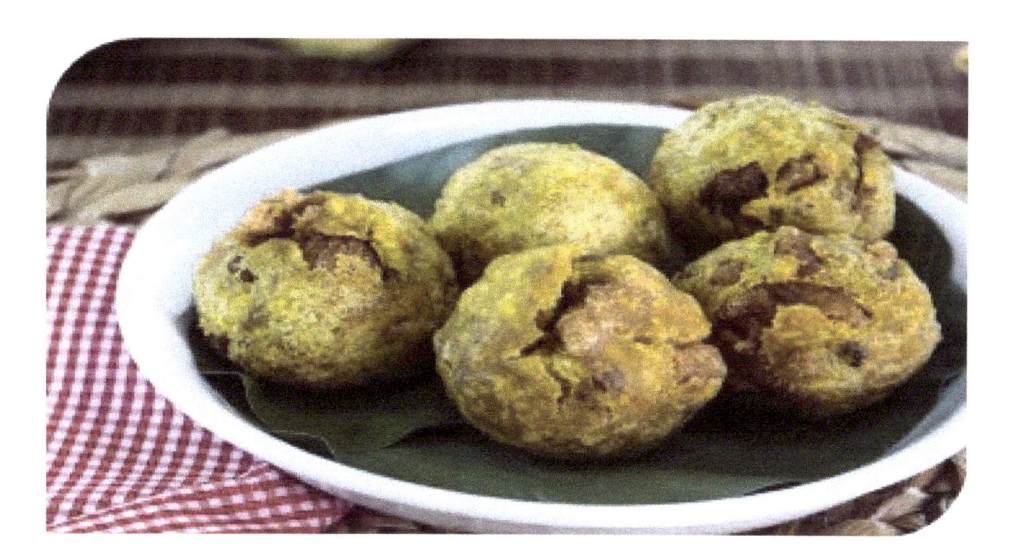

HEALTHY

Ingredients

- 2 ripe bananas
- Bacon
- cheese
- Olive oil
- Salt
- Pepper

Steps to Cook

1. Place the bananas cut in half to cook in water for 25 minutes and keep Cut the bacon into small pieces on a plate, add a splash of olive oil, salt and pepper to taste, place them separately in the fryer for 7 minutes at 1800C. At the end of the time, the pork rinds are turned and put another 7 minutes at 180ºC.

2. The first banana is taken, placed on top of a bag, covered with the same bag and crushed with a plate

3. The greaves are placed in the middle and with the bag they are closed giving the shape, this is done with each banana. Then the armed marranitas are placed in the fryer again with the same oil that released the pork rinds previously for 13 minutes at 180ºC.

4. To finish, place a slice of cheese and put another 5 minutes at 180ºC.

Nutritional Information

- Calories: 94
- Carbohydrates: 20g
- Fat: 0.3g
- Protein: 1.2g
- Sugar: 14g
- Cholesterol: 0mg

Air Fryer Cookbook

Chinese Bakery

• Servings: 8 • Preparation time: 1h 5 minutes • Cook time: 15 minutes •

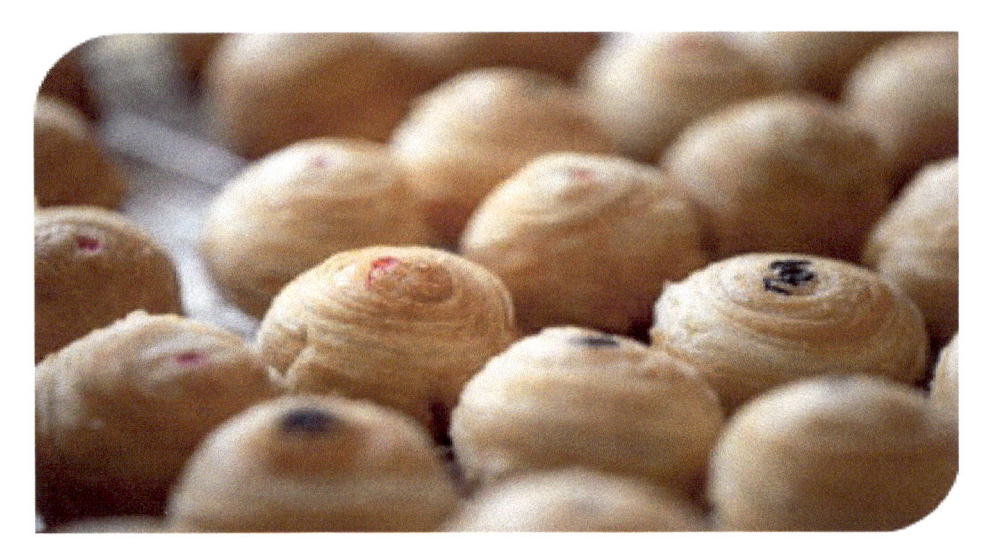

TASTY

Ingredients

- 6 ½ oz. warm milk
- ½ pound common wheat flour
- 2 tbsp sugar
- 1 tbsp of liquid butter
- ½ tbsp dry yeast of bakery
- ¼ tbsp of salt

Steps to Cook

1. Dissolve the yeast in the milk well in a glass together of sugar and cover. Let it ferment a little for 10 or 15 minutes. It looks like a foamy sponge, rather liquid.

2. Put the fermented mixture of the milk with the yeast, the liquid butter, the flour and the salt in the bowl in this order. Program dough menu. When it finishes kneading remove it from the bowl. Make a ball; brush it with a little oil and cover with a rag or plastic wrap. Let stand to ferment until double the volume.

3. When the dough is fermented degas it and with a rolling pin flatten the dough that you will make it with a thickness of 1 cm. The dough will be square.

4. Brush with oil and roll it up. Close the roll well and cut 8 pieces. With a piece of baking paper under each one you et rise make sure that they take the final shape. Put them in the air fryer for 15 minutes at 150ºC. Let cool on a rack. When they are cold, fry 1 minute on each side until they are golden brown.

Nutritional Information

- Calories: 1107
- Fat: 34g
- Protein: 55g
- Carbohydrates: 160g
- Sugar: 24g
- Cholesterol: 300mg

Potato Salad With Tuna

• Servings: 4 • Preparation time: 5 minutes • Cook time: 40 minutes •

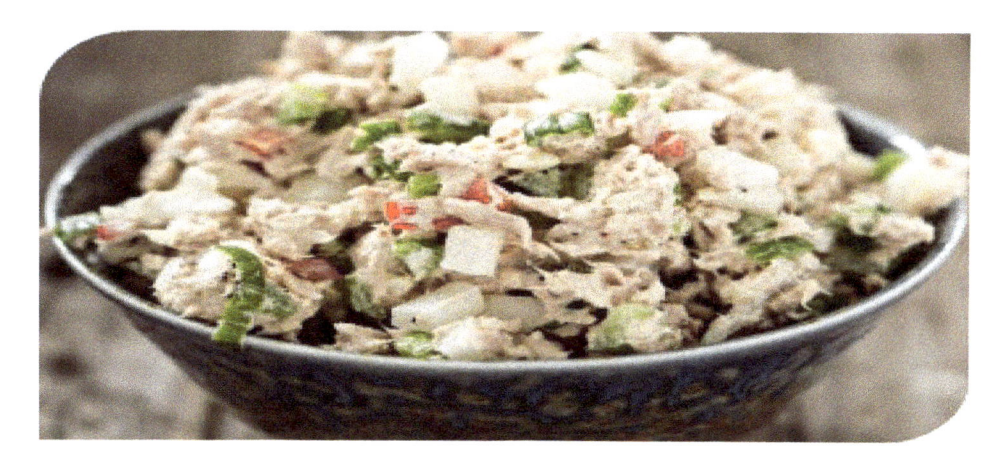

EXUBERANT

Ingredients

- 3 red roasting peppers
- 6 medium potatoes
- 2 small cans of tuna
- Extra virgin olive oil
- Salt
- Sherry vinager

Steps to Cook

1. Put boil the potatoes, cover them with water and add a little salt. When they are ready, drain and let cool.

2. Peel the potatoes, cut into slice and place on a tray or platter. Put the peppers on the oven tray, add salt and extra virgin olive oil.

3. Take to the air fryer, 170ºC, about 40 minutes or so. Take out when you see that the peppers are roasted.

4. Chill, peel and cut into strips.

5. Place the sliced peppers on top of the potatoes.

6. Put 3 parts extra virgin olive oil in a pot with 1 part sherry vinegar and salt.

7. Shake well and water the entire salad.

8. Drain the cans of tuna.

9. Put the tuna on top.

Nutritional Information

- Calories: 197
- Carbohydrates: 53g
- Fat: 1g
- Protein: 13g
- Sugar: 5g
- Cholesterol: 300mg

Air Fryer Cookbook

Gazpacho

• Servings: 4 • Preparation time: 2 minutes • Cook time: 23 minutes •

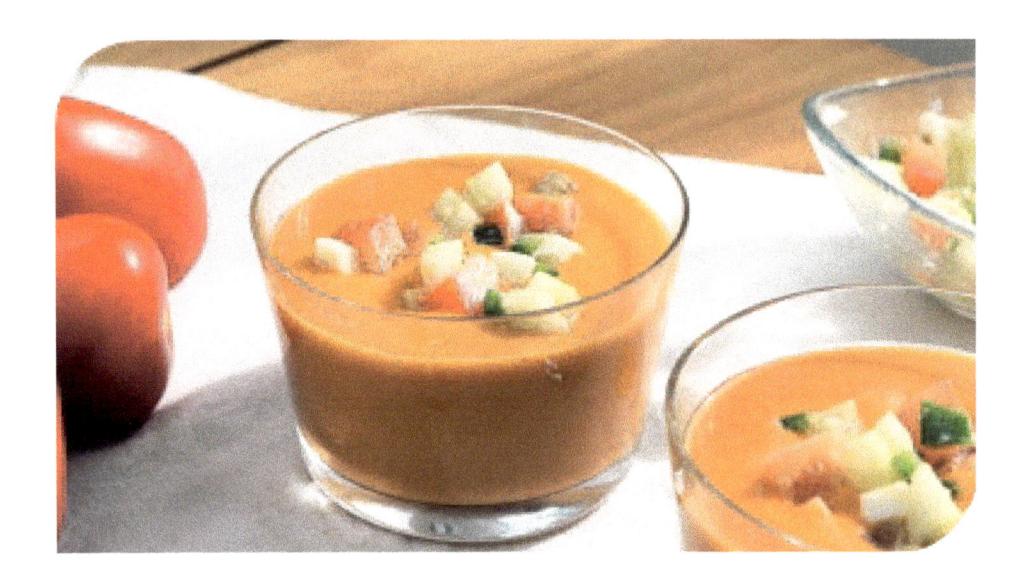

JUICY

Ingredients

- 1 cup cucumbers
- 2 cups of peeled tomatoes (canned or fresh)
- 3 garlic cloves
- ½ cup red pepper
- ½ cup red onion
- ½ cup of white wine vinegar
- 2 tsp olive oil
- 1 tbsp of ground pepper
- Salt

Steps to Cook

1. Cut the cucumber into 1 cm pieces. Chop the tomatoes. Chop the garlic, red pepper and onion into fine pieces.

2. Put all the ingredients in the air fryer, close the lid and select the soft soup program.

3. When the soup is done, pour it into a large bowl and let it cool for 3 hours in the fridge before serving.

Nutritional Information

- Calories: 100
- Carbohydrates: 16g
- Fat: 3g
- Protein: 1g
- Sugar: 10g
- Cholesterol: 0mg

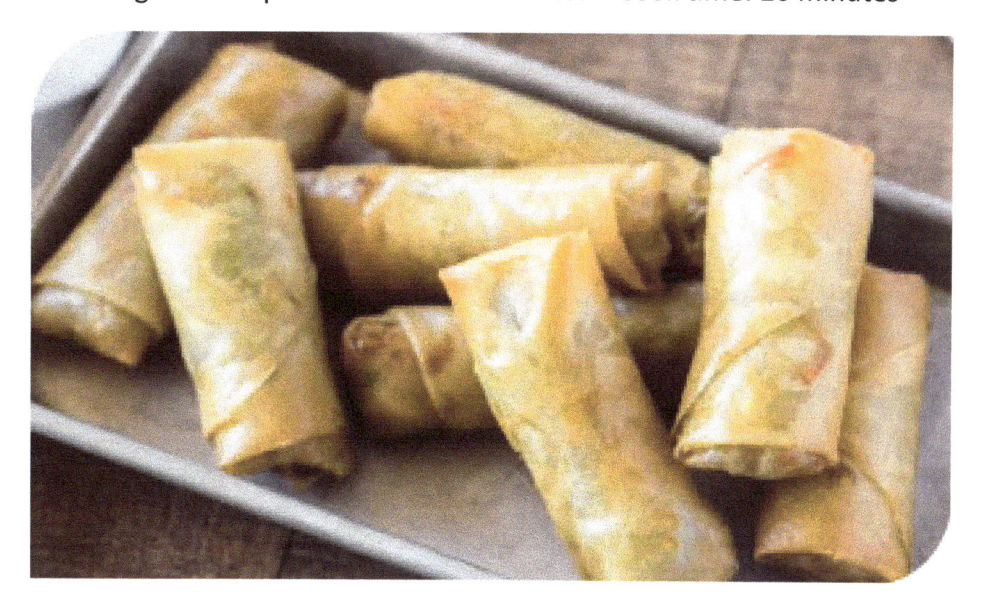

APPETIZING

Spring Rolls

• Servings: 4 • Preparation time: 10 minutes • Cook time: 20 minutes •

Ingredients

- ½ lb of minced pork
- 1 lb of white cabbage
- 1 onion
- 1 carrots
- 4 tbsp soy sauce
- Olive oil
- Salt
- 8 sheets of rice

Steps to Cook

1. Chop the onion, carrot and white cabbage. Put in the Wok a base of extra virgin olive oil. Add the vegetables that you have chopped and sauté.

2. Let the vegetables simmer over low heat.

3. Add the minced meat and season with salt and pepper. Braise well until the meat is cooked.

4. Add the soy sauce. Stir well and let it evaporate all the liquid it has. Let the filling cool down.

5. Hydrate the rice sheets until they are manageable; follow the directions on the package.

6. Spread on the work table. Spread the filling between the rice sheets. Tie the rolls.

7. Put in the air fryer, 180ºC for about 20 minutes.

Nutritional Information

- Calories: 326
- Carbohydrates: 12.1g
- Fat: 25.2g
- Protein: 13.4g
- Sugar: 0.5g
- Cholesterol: 10mg

Vegetables And Crispy Cheese Cubes

• Servings: 4 • Preparation time: 5 minutes • Cook time: 3-5 minutes •

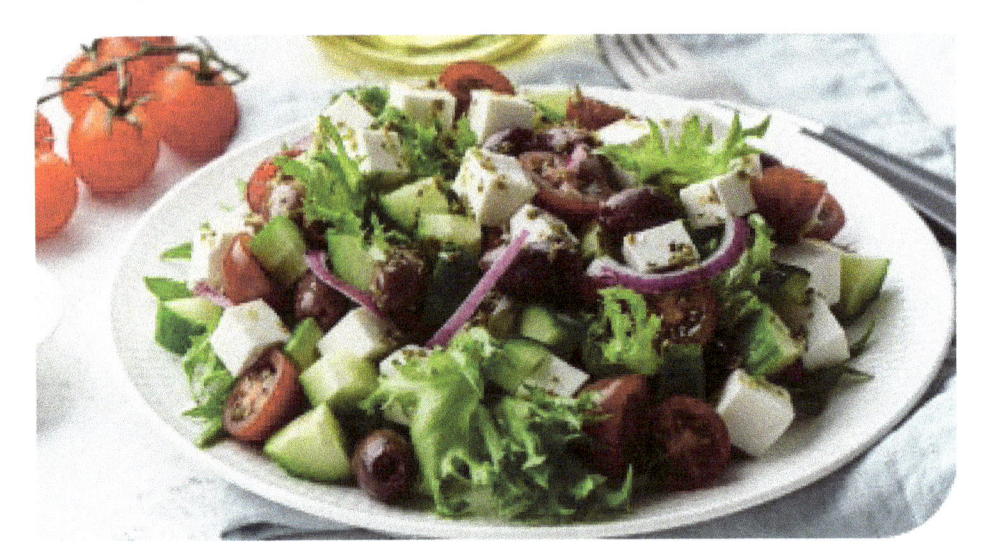

HEALTHY

Ingredients

- 1 romaine lettuce
- 2 or 3 tomatoes
- 8 cherry tomatoes
- 1 avocado
- 12 units of crispy cheese
- Extra virgin olive oil
- Salt
- Sherry vinager
- Reduction of Pedro Jimenez

Steps to Cook

1. Cut the lettuce, wash and dry.
2. Place the lettuce in a large salad bowl.
3. Chop the tomatoes and add them to the lettuce.
4. Spread the cherrys over the salad.
5. Peel the avocado and chop.
6. Spread the avocado over the salad.
7. Cook the crispy cheese in the Air fryer at 150ºC for 3 minutes.
8. Add a little salt, sherry vinegar and extra virgin olive oil to the salad

Nutritional Information

- Calories: 106
- Carbohydrates: 3.38g
- Fat: 7.28g
- Protein: 6.99g
- Sugar: 1.98g
- Cholesterol: 119mg

Meat Budin

• Servings: 6 • Preparation time: 10 minutes • Cook time: 12minutes •

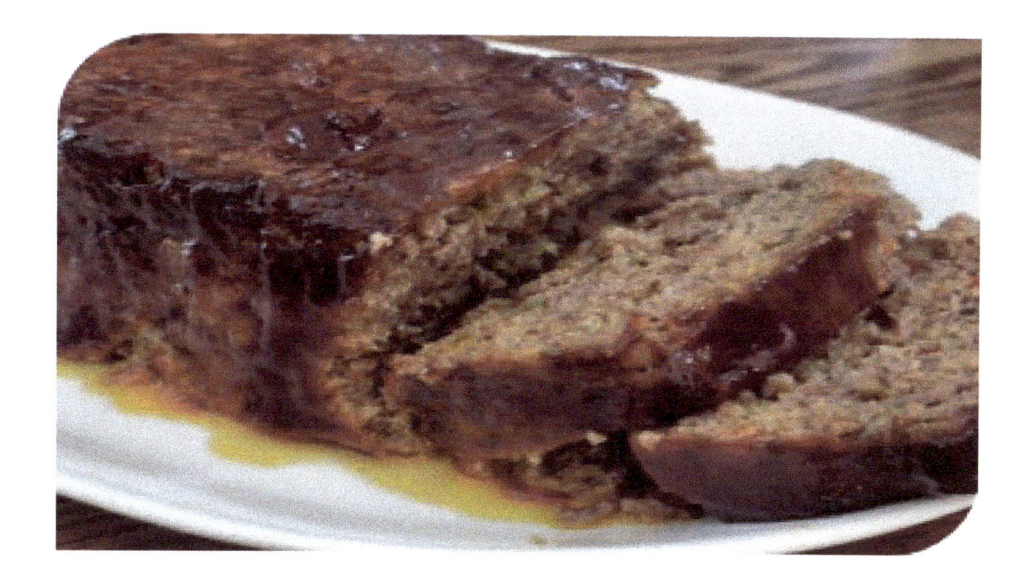

PALATABLE

Ingredients

- 1 lb lean ground beef
- 1 lightly beaten egg
- 3 tbsp of breadcrumbs
- 1 ½ oz. of finely chopped salami or chorizo
- 1 small onion, finely chopped
- 1 tbsp of fresh thyme
- Freshly ground pepper
- 2 mushrooms in thick slices
- 1 tbsp of olive oil

Steps to Cook

1. Preheat the air fryer to 200°C.

2. Mix the ground beef in a bowl with the egg, breadcrumbs, salami, onion, thyme, 1 teaspoon of salt and a generous amount of pepper. Love everything well.

3. Transfer the minced meat to the tray or platter and smooth the top. Place the mushrooms pressing a little and cover the top with olive oil.

4. Place the tray or platter in the basket and insert it in the air fryer. Set the timer to 25 minutes and grill the meat pudding until it is nice toasted and well done.

5. Let the pudding sit for at least 10 minutes before serving. Then cut it into wedges. It is delicious with chips and salad.

Nutritional Information

- Calories: 191
- Carbohydrates: 52g
- Fat: 9g
- Protein: 4g
- Sugar: 1g
- Cholesterol: 300mg

Air Fryer Cookbook

Potatoes With Sauce

• Servings: 4 • Preparation time: 5 minutes • Cook time: 10-15 minutes •

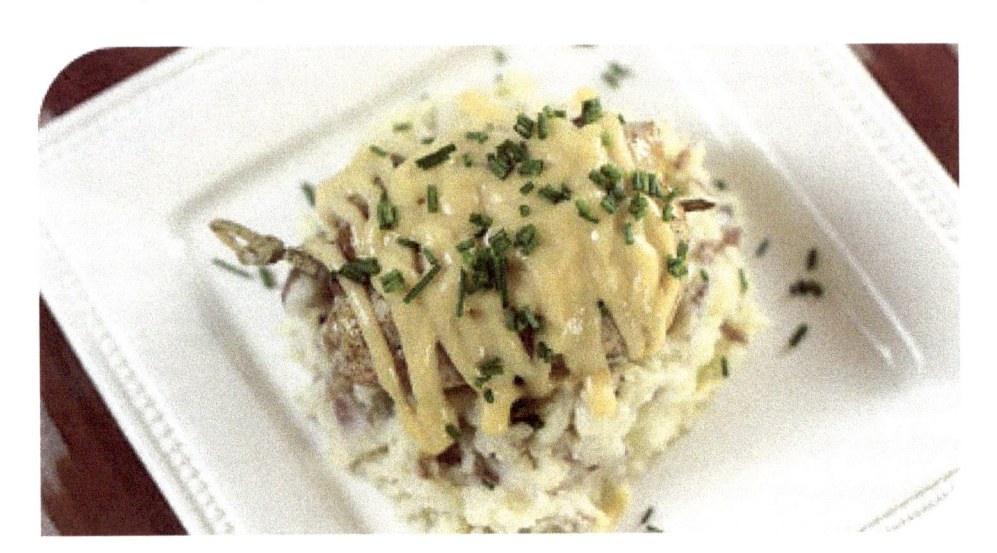

EASY & QUICK

Ingredients

- 2 lbs of potatoes
- 1 roasted chicken breast
- 1 cup of cream
- 1 tbsp of lemon juice
- 4 ½ oz. of mayonnaise
- 1 tbsp garlic powder
- 1 tbsp onion powder
- Salt
- Ground pepper
- Grated cheese, mine four grated cheeses

Steps to Cook

1. Fry the potatoes with the cane in abundant extra virgin olive oil.

2. Put the fried potatoes on a tray.

3. While the potatoes are frying, put the cream in a bowl, heat it in the microwave for 1 minute and add a tablespoon of lemon juice. Let it rest for 15 minutes.

4. After 15 minutes, add the mayonnaise, salt, ground pepper, garlic powder and onion powder to the bowl. Stir well and test to rectify any ingredient if necessary.

5. On the fried potatoes put the sauce well distributed, and also the cheese.

6. On the cheese we distribute the roasted and minced chicken.

7. Take to the air fryer for 5-10 minutes at 180ºC.

Nutritional Information

- Calories: 286.3
- Carbohydrates: 22.6g
- Fat: 3.3g
- Protein: 39.5g
- Sugar: 1.3g
- Cholesterol: 96.7mg

Prawns Orly

• Servings: 4 • Preparation time: 5 minutes • Cook time: 5-10 minutes •

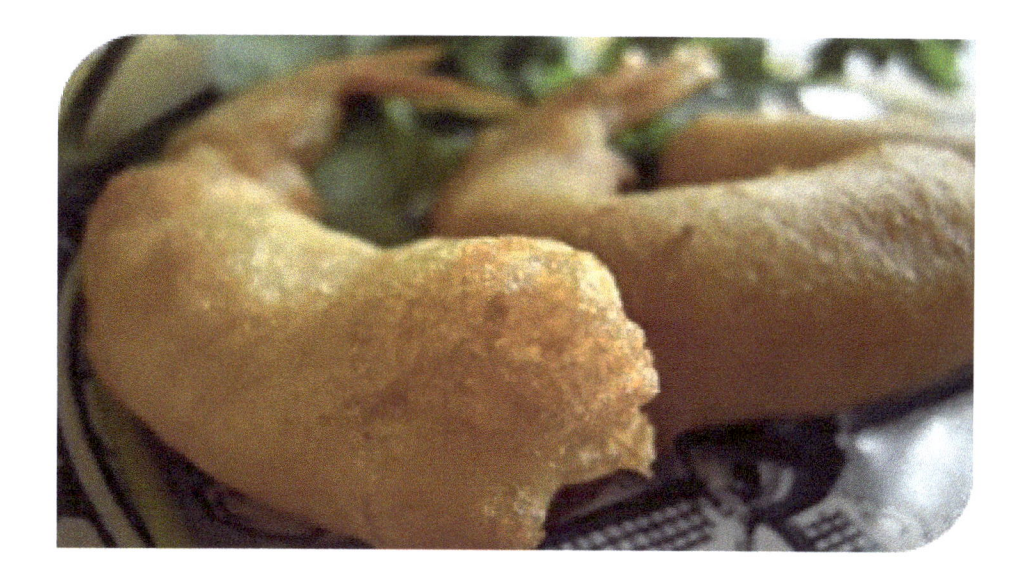

BUDGET FRIENDLY

Ingredients

- 24 white prawns
- 5 oz. of common flour
- 1/3 oz. cornstarch
- ¼ cup beer
- ½ cup sparkling water
- 1 egg
- 1 tsp of yeast
- Salt
- Extra virgin olive oil

optional: a little saffron

Steps to Cook

1. Peel the prawns leaving only the final tail, leave filmed in the fridge.

2. On the other hand we prepare the dough to coat the prawns, beating the yolk with the flour, beer, sparkling water, yeast and a little salt.

3. We mount the white to the point of snow and mix them with the rest of the dough, with enveloping movements so that as little air as possible is lost, and let it rest in the fridge for an hour.

4. Salt the prawns one by one and pass them through the mixture, automatically fry them in a saucepan or deep fryer at 180ºC until they begin to brown.

5. Drain them well of oil, pass them through kitchen paper and serve them quickly.

Nutritional Information

- Calories: 105
- Carbohydrates: 0.9g
- Fat: 1.72g
- Protein: 20.14g
- Sugar: 0g
- Cholesterol: 151mg

Air Fryer Cookbook

Ratatouille

• Servings: 2 • Preparation time: 5 minutes • Cook time: 15 minutes •

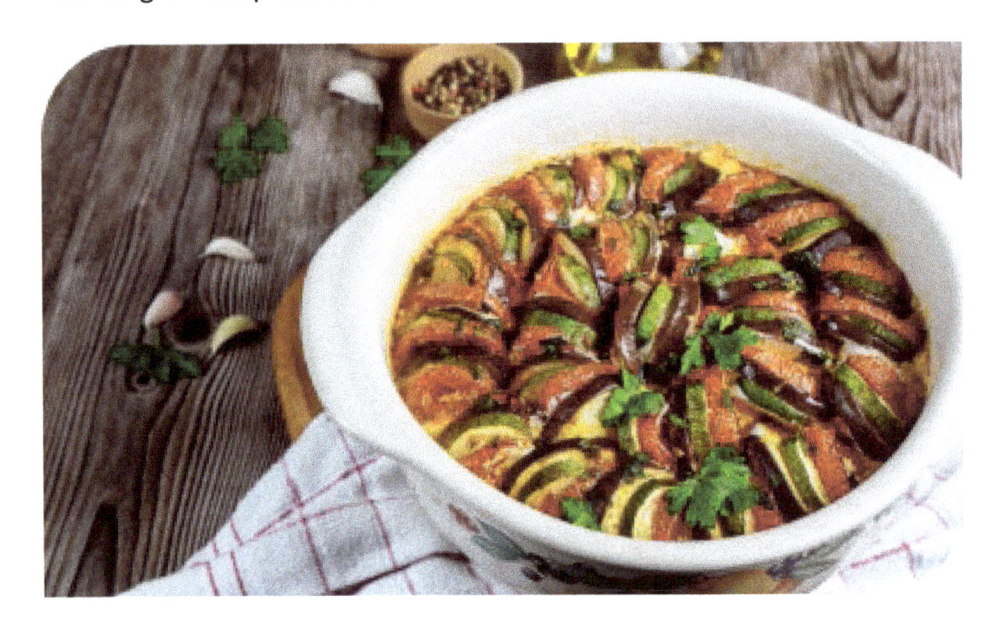

HEALTHY

Ingredients

- ½ lb zucchini and eggplant
- 1 yellow bell pepper
- 2 tomatoes
- 1 onion, peeled
- 1 garlic clove, crushed
- 2 tsp dried Provencal herbs
- Freshly ground black pepper
- 1 tbsp of olive oil

Steps to Cook

1. Preheat the air fryer to 200°C.

2. Cut the zucchini, eggplant, bell pepper, tomatoes, and onion into 2 cm cubes.

3. Mix the vegetables in a bowl with the garlic, the Provencal herbs, ½ teaspoon of salt and pepper to taste. Also add a tablespoon of olive oil.

4. Put the bowl in the basket and put it in the air fryer. Set the timer to 15 minutes and cook the ratatouille. Stir vegetables once while cooking.

5. Serve the ratatouille with fried meat like a steak or a cutlet.

Nutritional Information

- Calories: 154
- Carbohydrates: 11.94g
- Fat: 12.05g
- Protein: 1.69g
- Sugar: 5.22g
- Cholesterol: 0mg

Rösti

• Servings: 4 • Preparation time: 10 minutes • Cook time: 20 minutes •

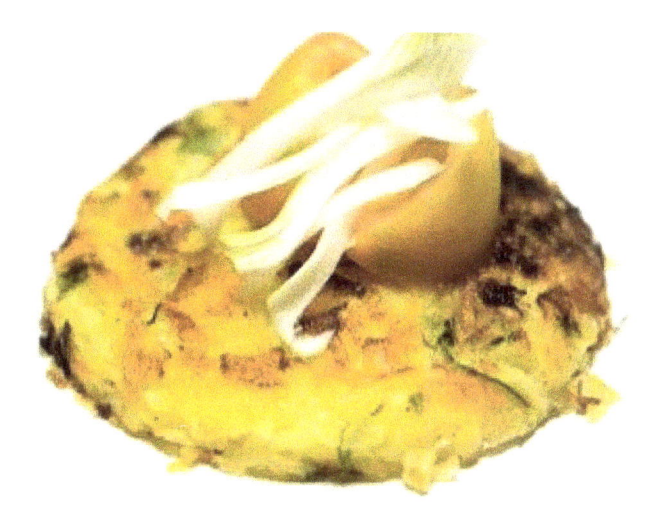

Ingredients

- ½ lb g peeled white potatoes
- 1 tbsp chives, finely chopped
- Freshly ground black pepper
- 1 tbsp of olive oil
- 2 tbsp of sour cream
- 3 ½ oz. smoked salmon

Steps to Cook

1. Preheat the air fryer to 180°C. Grate the thick potatoes in a bowl and add three quarters of the chives and salt and pepper to taste. Mix it well.

2. Grease the pizza pan with olive oil and distribute the potato mixture evenly throughout the pan. Press the grated potatoes against the pan and smear the top of the potato pie with olive oil.

3. Place the pizza tray in the fryer basket and insert it into the air fryer. Set the timer to 15 minutes and fry the rösti until it has a nice brownish color on the outside and is soft and well done on the inside.

4. Cut the rösti into 4 quarters and place each quarter on a plate. Garnish with a tablespoon of sour cream and place the salmon slices on the plate next to the rösti. Spread the rest of the chives on the sour cream and add a touch of ground pepper.

Nutritional Information

- Calories: 190
- Carbohydrates: 30g
- Fat: 6g
- Protein: 2g
- Sugar: 2g
- Cholesterol: 57mg

Salmon quiche

• Servings: 4 • Preparation time: 5 minutes • Cook time: 20 minutes •

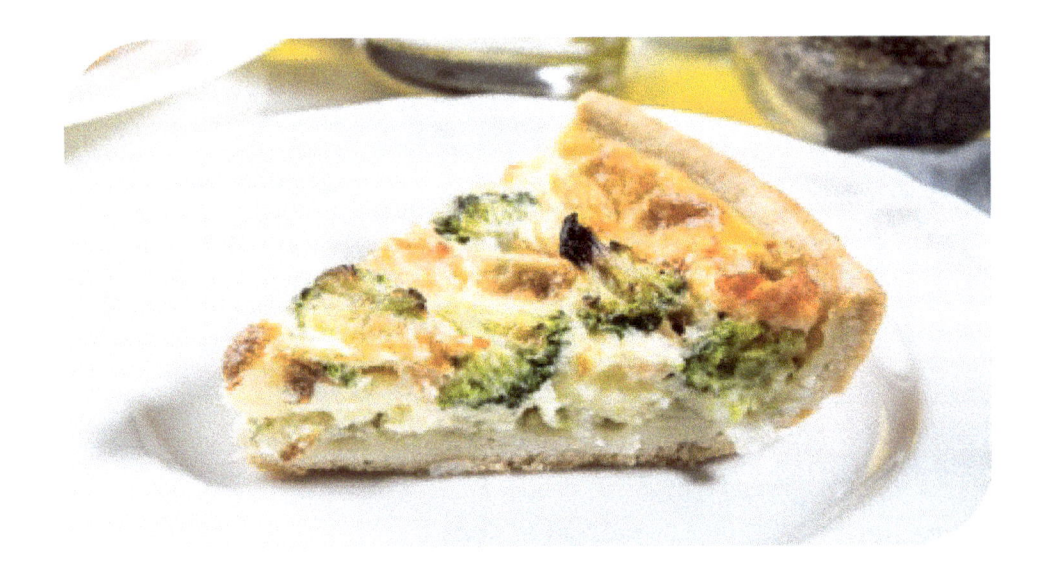

CREAMY

Ingredients

- 1/3 lb salmon fillets, diced
- ½ tbsp of lemon juice
- Freshly ground black pepper
- 3 ½ oz of flour
- 2 oz. diced cold butter
- 2 eggs + 1 egg yolk
- 3 tbsp of milk cream
- ½ tbsp mustard
- 1 chive cut into 1 cm slices

Steps to Cook

1. Preheat the air fryer to 180°C. Mix the salmon pieces with the lemon juice and add salt and pepper to taste. Let it rest. In a bowl, mix the flour with the butter, the egg yolk and 1 and a half tablespoons of cold water and knead until you get a uniform ball.

2. On a floured work surface, roll out the dough to an 18 cm circle. Place the circle of dough on the quiche tray and press well around the edges. Trim the dough off the edge of the tray or let it protrude along the edges.

3. Beat the eggs lightly with the cream and mustard and add salt and pepper to taste. Pour this mixture on the quiche tray and then place the pieces of salmon on it. Distribute the chives evenly over the contents of the tray. Put in the air fryer to 20 minutes. Ready!

Nutritional Information

- Calories: 287.2
- Carbohydrates: 11.4
- Fat: 13g
- Protein: 29.5g
- Sugar: 0.2g
- Cholesterol: 212.4mg

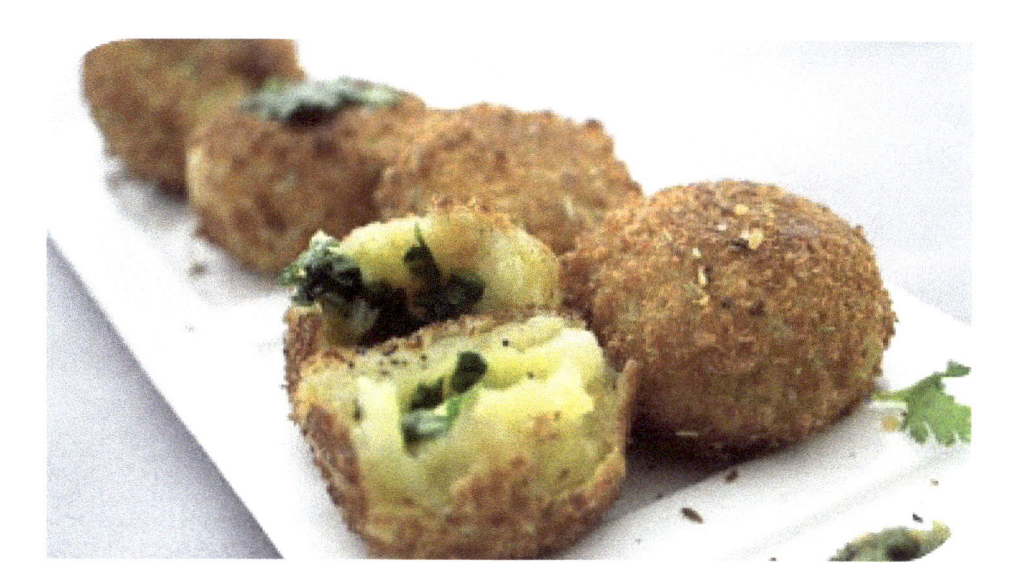

TOOTHSOME

Cottage Cheese Balls With Basil

• Servings: 4 • Preparation time: 5 minutes • Cook time: 8 minutes •

Ingredients

- ½ lb of cottage cheese
- 2 tbsp of flour
- 1 egg, separated
- Freshly ground pepper
- ½ oz. basil, chopped
- 1 tbsp chives, chopped
- 1 tbsp grated orange zest
- 3 slices of hardened white bread
- 1 tbsp of olive oil

Steps to Cook

1. Mix the cottage cheese in a bowl with the flour and the egg yolk, 1 teaspoon of salt and freshly ground pepper. Whisk the basil, chives and orange zest with the mixture.

2. Divide the mixture into 20 equal portions and create balls with wet hands. Let the balls sit for a while.

3. Grate the bread into thin pieces with the food processor and mix it with olive oil. Pour the mixture into a deep plate. Beat the egg in another deep plate.

4. Preheat the air fryer to 200°C.

5. Carefully coat the cottage cheese balls in the egg white, and then roll them over the breadcrumbs.

6. Put 10 balls in the basket and put it in the air fryer. Set the timer to 8 minutes. Bake them until golden brown. Bake the rest in the same way.

Nutritional Information

- Calories: 43.1
- Carbohydrates: 10.5g
- Fat: 1.1g
- Protein: 2.8g
- Sugar: 3g
- Cholesterol: 0.6mg

Stew Broth Croquettes

• Servings: 4 • Preparation time: 5 minutes • Cook time: 15 minutes •

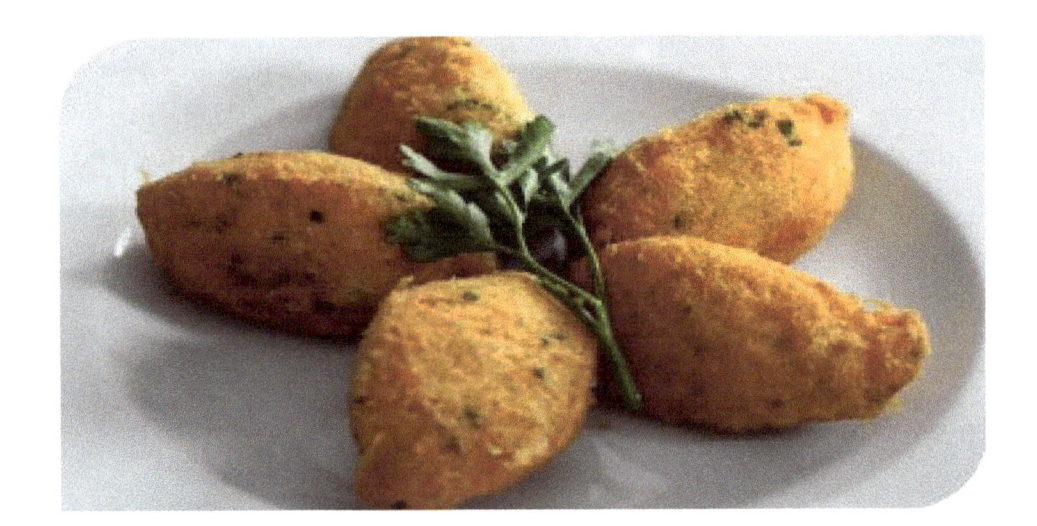

DELICIOUS

Ingredients

- ½ Meat (beef)
- 2 ½ oz. extra virgin oil
- 1 onion
- ½ lb of wheat flour
- 1 lb of broth
- Nutmeg
- Salt
- Ground pepper
- To bread the croquettes, flour, beaten egg, breadcrumbs
- Extra virgin olive oil to paint the croquettes

Steps to Cook

1. Put in the cuisine the accessory of the ultrablade mincer. Add the extra virgin olive oil and the onion cut into quarters. Select 5 minutes, 100ºC and speed 6. Add the flour and select 3 minutes, 100ºC and speed 4. Add the broth, season and add a little nutmeg. Select 10 seconds, speed 8. Add the minced and boneless meat. Select 10 minutes, 130 degrees temperature, speed 4.

2. Remove the dough to a tray and let cool.

3. Once the dough is cold, make the croquettes.

4. We go through flour, beaten egg and breadcrumbs.

5. When frying, put the croquettes in the basket of the Air fryer and paint them with extra virgin olive oil. Do not pile up.

6. Select 180ºC, 20 minutes.

Nutritional Information

- Calories: 195.6
- Carbohydrates: 2.2g
- Fat: 15g
- Protein: 11.2g
- Sugar: 0.2g
- Cholesterol: 69.1mg

Guava Empanadas With Cheese

• Servings: 4 • Preparation time: 5 minutes • Cook time: 40-45 minutes •

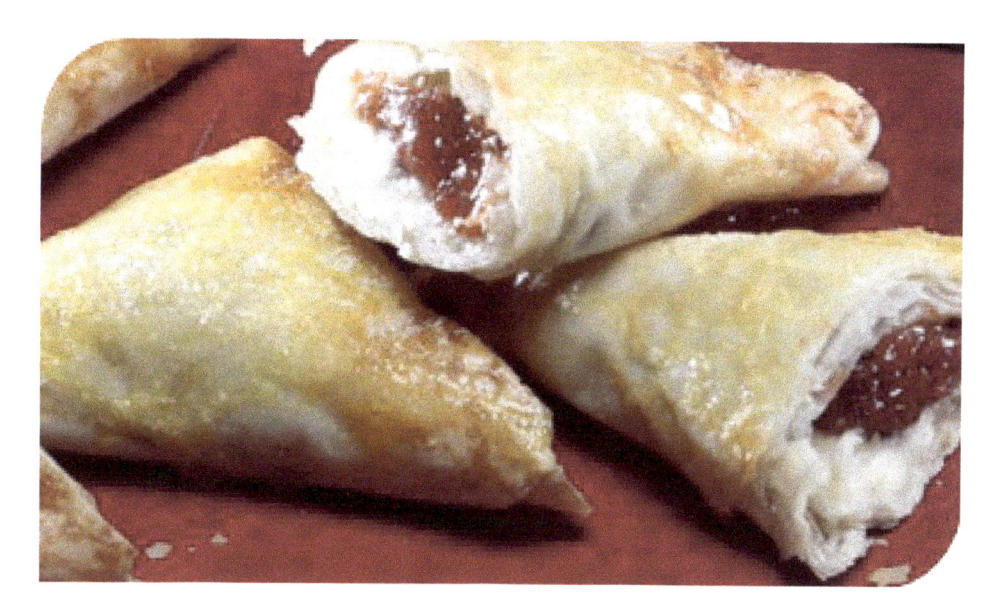

FRUITY

Ingredients

- enough water
- 1 lb of guava
- 2 piloncillos
- ¼ cups of water
- 1 cinnamon stick
- enough sugar to spread
- enough flour to spread
- enough of puff pastry
- ½ cups cream cheese, diced
- enough egg, to varnish

Steps to Cook

1. Preheat the air fryer to 200°C. Cook the guavas for 10 minutes in boiling water until they are slightly soft, drain and reserve. Remove the seeds. Place the piloncillo in a saucepan with ¼ cup of water and cinnamon, cook for 10 minutes until you get a honey, add the guavas and cook until it has a thick consistency and slightly crumble. Reserve.

2. On a clean surface sprinkle sugar, spread the puff pastry to 3 mm thick with the help of a rolling pin and if necessary add a little flour. Cut in circles with the help of a 10 cm diameter cutter.

3. Fill the puff pastry discs with the guava and add the cream cheese squares, close with the help of a fork. Put in the air fryer for 20 minutes.

Nutritional Information

- Calories: 254.5
- Carbohydrates: 2.6g
- Fat: 16.2g
- Protein: 6.1g
- Sugar: 1g
- Cholesterol: 76.3mg

Chapter 5

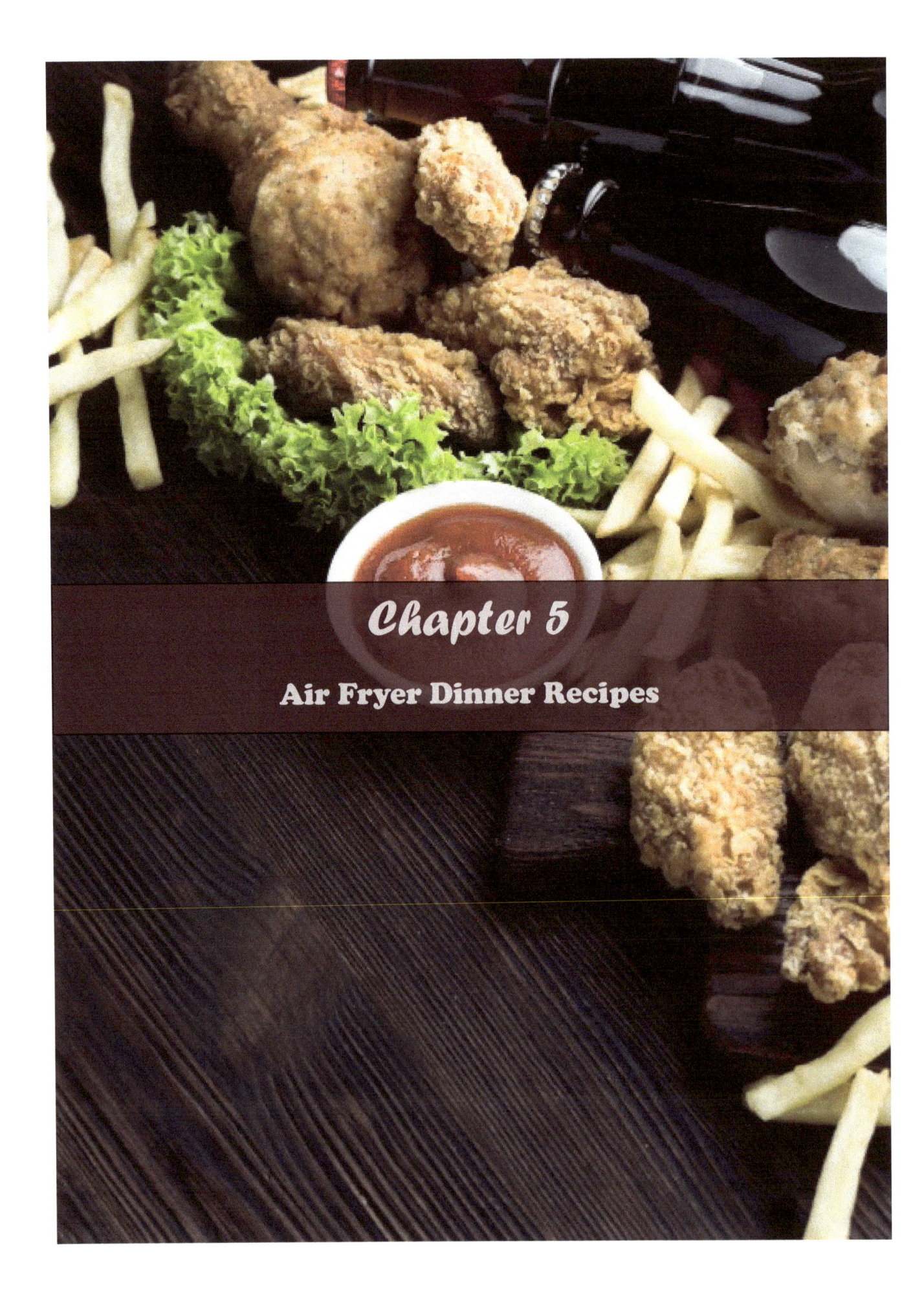

Air Fryer Dinner Recipes

Chocolate Express

• Servings: 6 • Preparation time: 10 minutes • Cook time: 15 minutes •

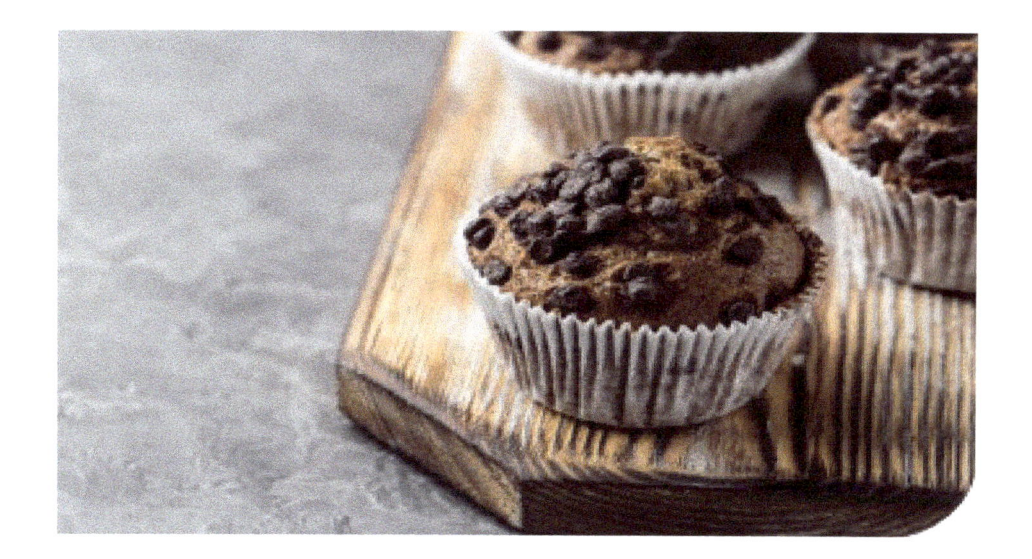

CHOCOLATY

Ingredients

- 4 ¼ oz. flour
- 2 oz. cocoa powder
- 150 g light brown sugar
- 5 ¼ oz. baking powder
- ½ tsp coffee powder
- ½ tsp of baking soda
- ¼ tsp of salt
- 1 large egg
- ½ cup milk
- 1 tsp of vanilla extract
- 1 tsp apple cider vinegar
- 80 ml of vegetable oil
- Non-stick spray oil

Steps to Cook

1. Mix together the flour, cocoa powder, sugar, baking powder, espresso powder, baking soda, and salt in a large bowl.

2. Whisk together the egg, milk, vanilla, vinegar, and oil in a separate bowl.

3. Mix the wet ingredients into the dry ingredients until well combined.

4. Grease the muffin tins with cooking spray and pour the mixture until they are full to ¾.

5. Select Preheat, in the air fryer adjust the temperature to 150°C.

6. Carefully place the muffin tins in the preheated air fryer. You may need to work in parts.

7. Select Desserts, set the time to 15 minutes.

Nutritional Information

- Calories: 690
- Carbohydrates: 79.2g
- Fat: 38g
- Protein: 9.9g
- Sugar: 15g
- Cholesterol: 125mg

Air Fryer Cookbook

Sweet Sponge Cake

• Servings:10• Preparation time: 10 minutes• Cook time: 50 minutes •

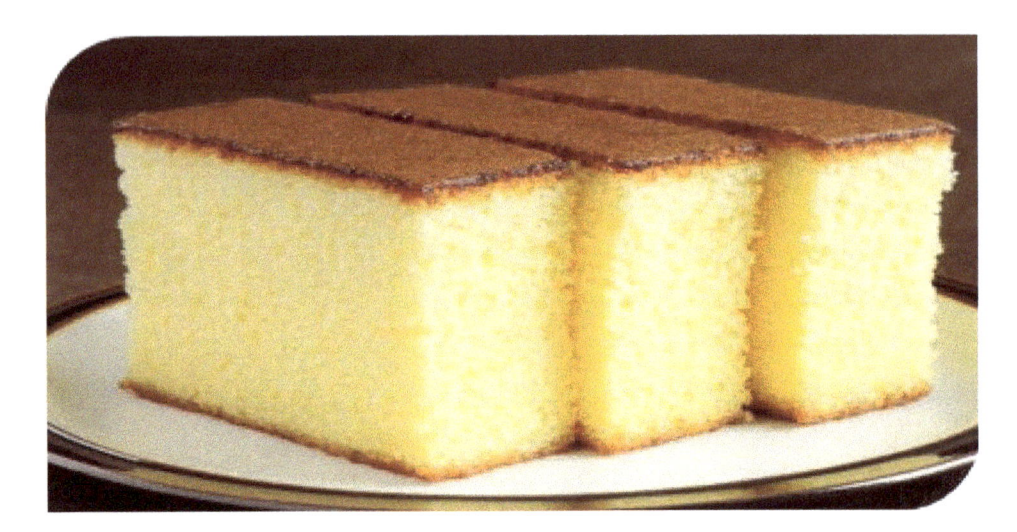

SPONGY

Ingredients

- ½ lb flour for
- yeast pastry
- ½ lb of sugar
- 3 medium eggs
- 3 tbsp olive oil
- Orange zest
- ¾ lb chopped pistachio
- 1 envelope of yeast

Steps to Cook

1. Separate the yolks from the eggs. Mount the egg whites until stiff with the mixer and gradually incorporate the sugar.

2. Mix until you get a thick white cream.

3. Separately, beat the yolks with the oil and the orange zest. Incorporate this mixture with the whites, mix in an enveloping way and finally incorporate the flour and yeast with a sieve. When everything is well mixed, add the pistachios. You can use a circular mold greased with oil and flour or kitchen paper that is more comfortable. Add the cake batter to the pan.

4. Preheat the Air fryer for a few minutes at 160ºC. Put the mold in the basket of the Air fryer and program the timer for about 30 minutes at 1600C temperature.

5. While it is cooking prepare the lemon cream.

6. To do this, gradually mix the white with the sugar, add the lemon juice and add the sour cream and mix until obtaining a thick cream and ready.

Nutritional Information

- Calories: 110
- Carbohydrates:23g
- Fat: 1g
- Protein: 2.1g
- Sugar: 14g
- Cholesterol: 39mg

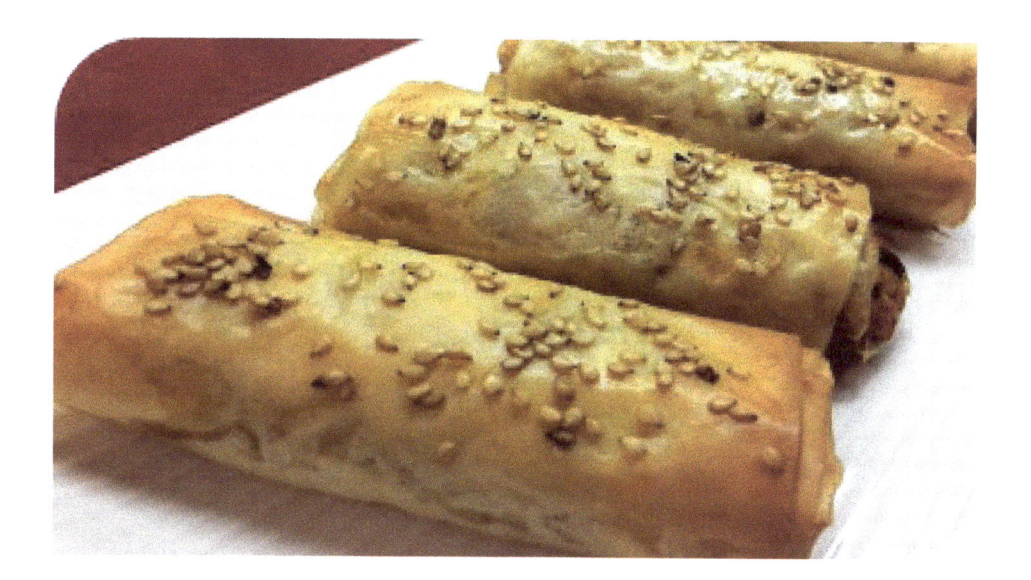

APPETIZING

Philo Pasta Rolls

• Servings: 4 • Preparation time: 5 minutes • Cook time: 20 minutes •

Ingredients

- 4 sheets of philo paste
- 2 small cans of tuna
- 1 onion
- 1 green pepper
- Fried tomato sauce
- 2 ½ oz. of white cabbage
- Extra virgin olive oil
- Salt
- Ground pepper

Steps to Cook

1. Put in a frying pan a bottom of extra virgin olive oil.

2. Add the onion, pepper and white cabbage, all very chopped. Begin to make the sofrito and I count we have the tender vegetables, we add the drained and crumbled tuna.

3. Link and add the tomato sauce, just enough to leave a thick and not very liquid dough.

4. Rectify with salt and let it cool down. Spread the sheets of philo paste and distribute the filling between them. Tie the rolls so that they are well sealed. Place on the appetizer tray of your air fryer.

5. Paint with a little extra virgin olive oil and a brush.

6. We select 20 minutes at 180ºC.

Nutritional Information

- Calories: 197
- Carbohydrates: 53g
- Fat: 1g
- Protein: 13g
- Sugar: 5g
- Cholesterol: 300mg

Air Fryer Cookbook

Mini Sausage Patty

• Servings: 4 • Preparation time: 2 minutes • Cook time: 23 minutes •

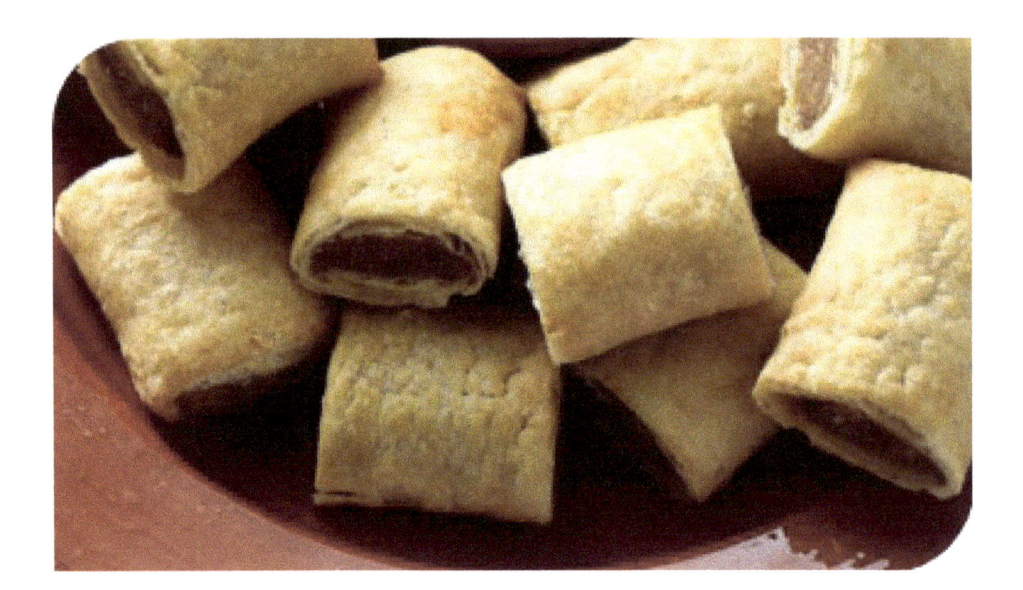

DELICIOUS

Ingredients

- 1 bottle of mini sausages (net weight 7 oz, approx. 20 sausages)
- 3 ½ oz. puff pastry ready to make (refrigerated or frozen, already thawed)
- 1 tbsp of fine mustard

Steps to Cook

1. Preheat the air fryer to 200°C.

2. Dry the sausages completely with kitchen paper with light touches.

3. Cut the puff pastry into strips of 5 x 1½ cm length and cover them with a thin layer of mustard.

4. Roll each sausage in a spiral into a puff pastry strip.

5. Place half of the sausage puffs in the basket and place it in the air fryer. Set the timer to 10 minutes. Bake until golden brown. Bake the rest of the puff pastry in the same way.

6. Serve them on a tray accompanied by a small plate of mustard.

Nutritional Information

- Calories: 150
- Carbohydrates: 1g
- Fat: 13g
- Protein: 6g
- Sugar: 0g
- Cholesterol: 275mg

Blueberry and Lemon Cake

• Servings: 4 • Preparation time: 5 minutes • Cook time: 5-10 minutes •

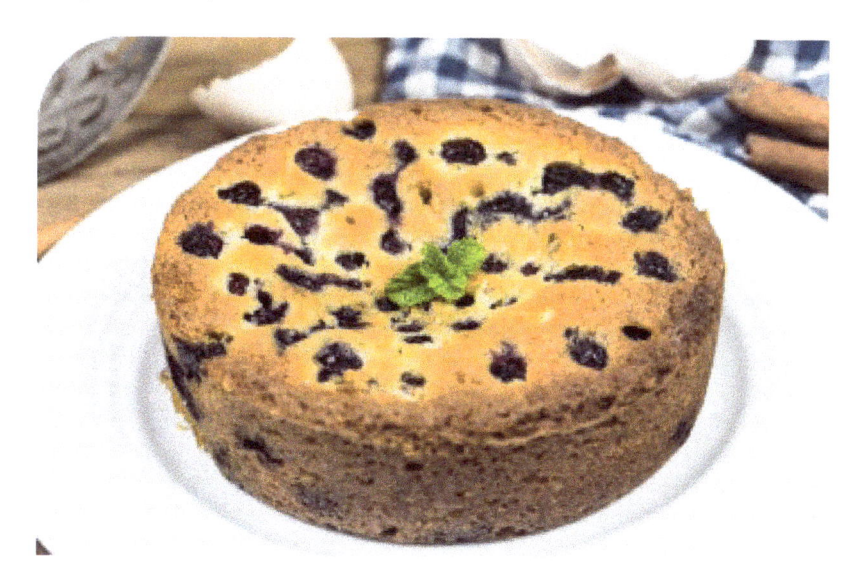

FLAVORSOME

Ingredients

- 1 tsp lemon juice
- 4 oz. coconut milk
- 4 ¼ oz. flour
- 1 ¼ tsp baking powder
- ½ tsp of baking soda
- ¼ tsp of salt
- 2 oz. granulated sugar
- ¼ oz. coconut oil
- 1 lemon, lemon zest
- 1 tsp of vanilla extract
- 2 oz. of fresh blueberries
- Non-stick spray oil

Steps to Cook

1. Combine lemon juice and coconut milk in a small bowl. Set aside. Mix the flour, baking powder, baking soda, and salt in a separate bowl and set aside.

2. Mix the sugar, coconut oil, lemon zest, and vanilla extract in an additional bowl. Then combine with the coconut-lemon mix and stir to combine.

3. Mix dry to wet ingredients gradually, until mixture is smooth. Gently lay out the blueberries.

4. Select Preheat, in the air fryer adjust the temperature to 150°C. Grease the muffin tins with cooking spray and pour the mixture until the cups are ¾.

5. Carefully place the muffin tins in the preheated air fryer. Select Desserts, set the time to 15 minutes.

....

Nutritional Information

- Calories: 326
- Carbohydrates: 12.1g
- Fat: 25.2g
- Protein: 13.4g
- Sugar: 0.5g
- Cholesterol: 10mg

Air Fryer Cookbook

Cachopo

• Servings:2• Preparation time: 5 minutes• Cook time: 25 minutes •

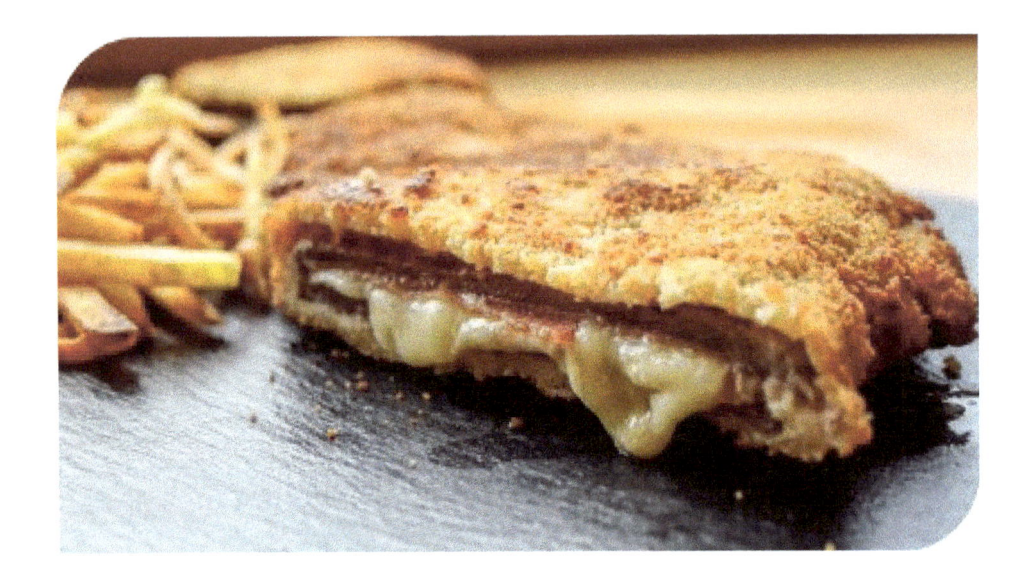

HEALTHY

Ingredients

- 4 beef fillets
- Cured ham slices
- Roasted peppers
- To bread flour, egg and breadcrumbs
- Extra virgin olive oil
- Salt
- Ground pepper

Steps to Cook

1. Season the fillets and fill with slices of cured ham and roasted red peppers.

2. Press well and go through flour, beaten egg and breadcrumbs to bread well.

3. Paint everything very well with extra virgin olive oil. Let it be well wet.

4. Place in the basket of the Air fryer and select 15 minutes at 160ºC and 10 more minutes at 180ºC.

5. When we see that they are well gilded on the outside, we take out.

Nutritional Information

- Calories: 164
- Carbohydrates: 12g
- Fat: 1g
- Protein: 24g
- Sugar: 0g
- Cholesterol: 300mg

Green Salad With Roasted Pepper

• Servings: 4 • Preparation time: 5 minutes • Cook time: 10 minutes •

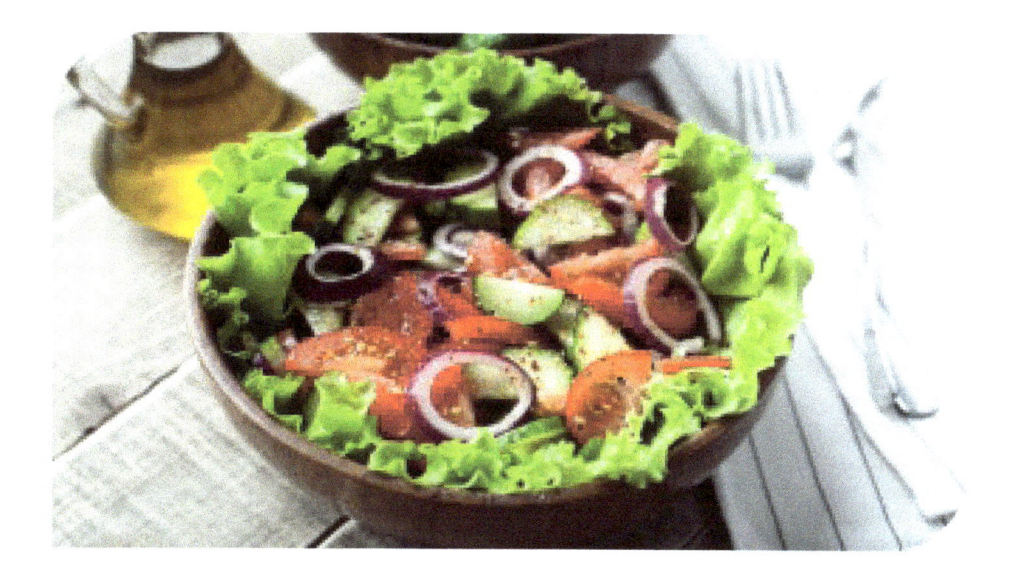

HEALTHY

Ingredients

- 1 red pepper
- 1 tbsp of lemon juice
- 3 tbsp of yogurt
- 2 tbsp of olive oil
- Freshly ground black pepper
- 1 romaine lettuce in wide strips
- 1 ½ oz. of arugula leaves

Steps to Cook

1. Preheat the air fryer to 200°C.

2. Put the bell pepper in the basket and put it in the air fryer. Set the timer to 10 minutes and grill the pepper until the skin is slightly burned.

3. Place the pepper in a bowl and cover it with a lid or with plastic wrap. Let it sit for 10 to 15 minutes.

4. Next, cut the pepper into four parts and remove the seeds and skin. Cut the pepper into strips.

5. Mix a dressing in a bowl with 2 tablespoons of the pepper juice, lemon juice, yogurt, and olive oil. Add pepper and salt to taste.

6. Pour the lettuce and arugula leaves into the dressing and garnish the salad with the pepper strips.

Nutritional Information

- Calories: 106
- Carbohydrates: 3.38g
- Fat: 7.28g
- Protein: 6.99g
- Sugar: 1.98g
- Cholesterol: 119mg

Garlic Mushrooms

• Servings:4• Preparation time: 2 minutes• Cook time: 20 minutes •

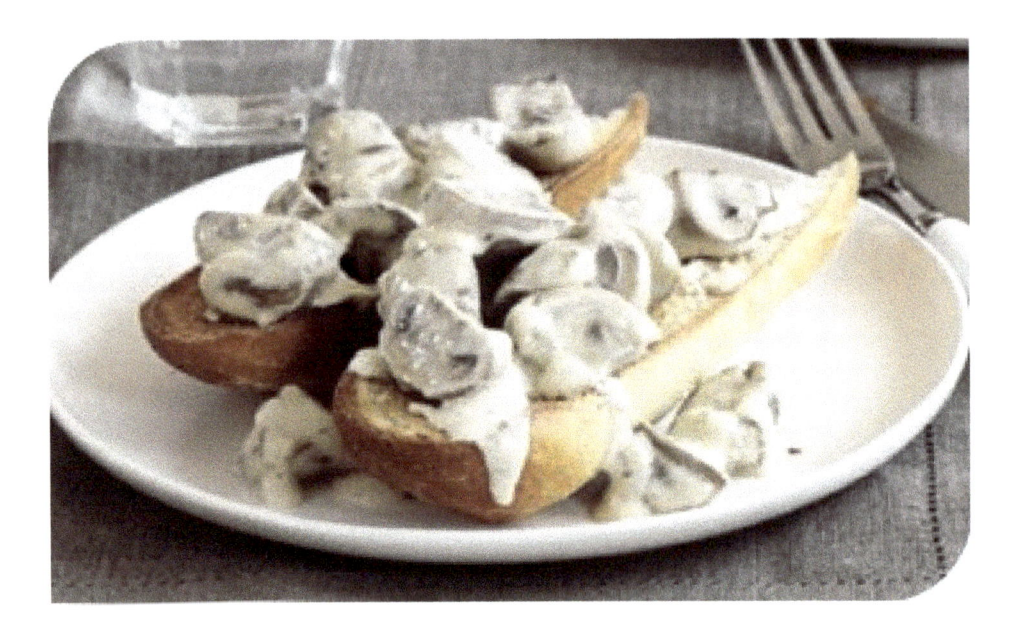

CRISPY

Ingredients

- 1 slice of white bread
- 1 garlic clove, crushed
- 1 tbsp of chopped parsley
- Freshly ground black pepper
- 1 tbsp of olive oil
- 12 mushrooms

Steps to Cook

1. Preheat the air fryer to 200°C.

2. Grate the slice of bread until it is fine in the food processor and mix it with the garlic, parsley and season to taste. Finally, pour in the olive oil.

3. Remove the stems from the mushrooms and fill the caps with the breadcrumbs.

4. Put the mushrooms in the basket and put it in the air fryer. Set the timer to 10 minutes. Bake until golden and crisp.

Nutritional Information

- Calories: 139
- Carbohydrates: 6.1g
- Fat: 11.6g
- Protein: 4.7g
- Sugar: 3.5g
- Cholesterol: 30.4mg

Chicken Salad

• Servings: 6 • Preparation time: 10 minutes • Cook time: 15 minutes •

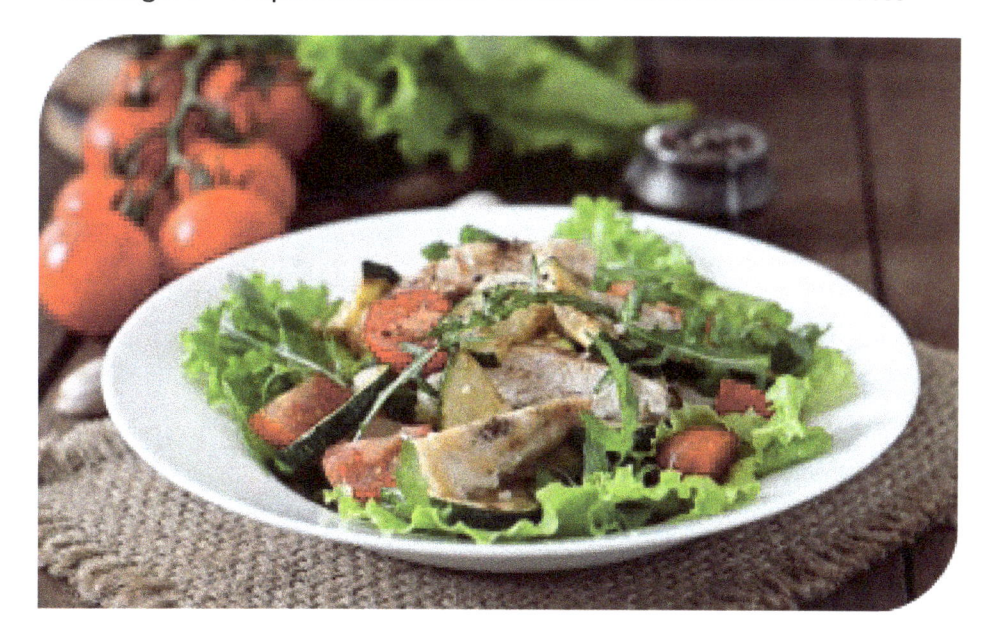

Ingredients

Vinaigrette: 1 tbsp of balsamic vinegar cream

- 2 tbsp sherry vinegar
- 2 tbsp of mustard
- 1 tsp salt
- Ground pepper
- Garlic powder
- 6 tbsp of virgin olive oil
- 1 romaine lettuce
- 1 can of sweet corn
- 12 pieces chicken
- A little grated

Steps to Cook

1. Put the vinaigrette ingredients in a pot and shake well.

2. Cut the lettuce and place in a salad bowl.

3. Put the breaded chicken pieces in the air fryer. Select 200ºC for 25 minutes. When it is ready, take it out and distribute.

4. Drain the sweet corn and add to the salad.

5. Add a little cheese, grated or diced.

6. Bathe the salad with the vinaigrette.

Nutritional Information

- Calories: 106
- Carbohydrates: 3.38g
- Fat: 7.28g
- Protein: 6.99g
- Sugar: 1.98g
- Cholesterol: 119mg

Air Fryer Cookbook

Crispy Potato Dices

• Servings:4• Preparation time: 5 minutes• Cook time: 15 minutes •

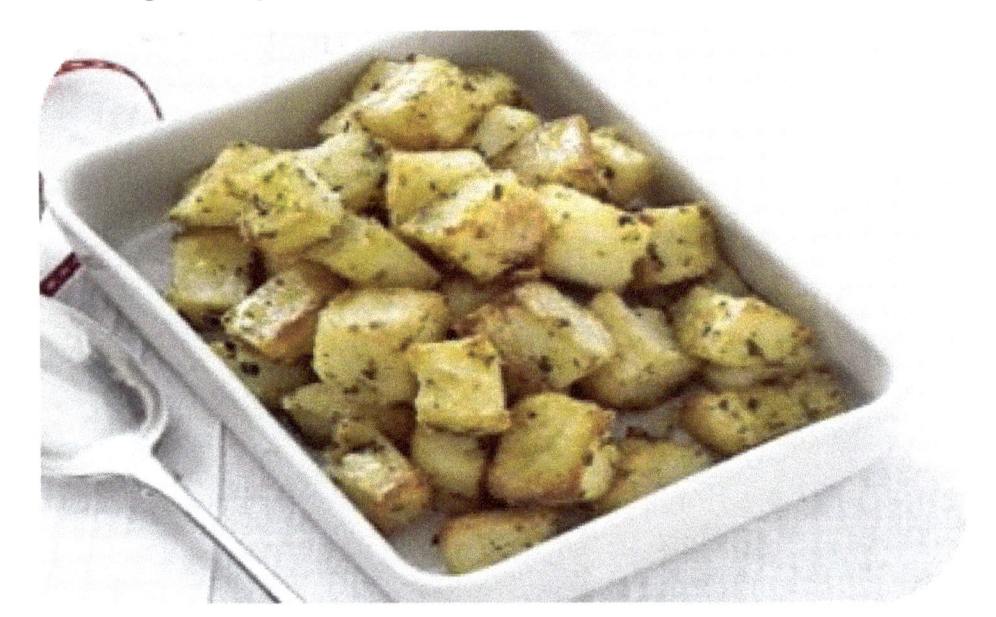

CRUNCHY

Ingredients

- 1 ½ lb of white potatoes
- 1 tbsp mild curry powder
- 1 tbsp of vegetable oil
- 1 small ripe mango, sliced (fresh or canned)
- 3 tsp of fresh coriander, finely chopped
- Juice and zest of half a lime
- Freshly ground black pepper

Steps to Cook

1. Preheat the air fryer to 1800C Peel the potatoes and cut them into cubes 2 cm wide. Soak the cubes in water for at least 30 minutes. Dry them well with kitchen paper.

2. Mix the curry powder and oil in a bowl and coat the potato cubes with this mixture. Place the dice in the fryer basket and insert it into the air fryer. Set the timer to 15 minutes and fry the dice until golden and ready to drink. Rotate them from time to time.

3. Meanwhile, beat the mango with the cilantro and the juice and the zest of the lime in a mixer and add salt and pepper to taste.

Nutritional Information

- Calories: 286.3
- Carbohydrates: 22.6g
- Fat: 3.3g
- Protein: 39.5g
- Sugar: 1.3g
- Cholesterol: 96.7mg

Fried Anchovies

• Servings: 4 • Preparation time: 10 minutes • Cook time: 20 minutes •

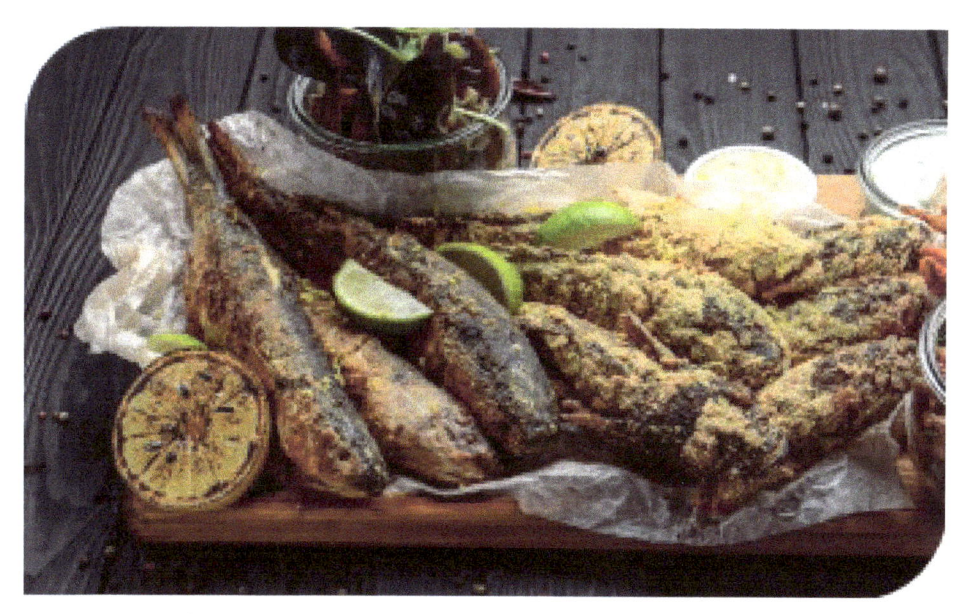

Ingredients

- 1 lb of anchovies
- Salt
- Flour
- Oil spray

Steps to Cook

1. Clean the anchovies. You can, if we want, open in half and remove the central spine.

2. Wash well, drain and put salt.

3. Pass the anchovies by flour and place them on a large tray so that they are separated from each other.

4. Spray with the oil bottle so that the oil is well distributed by all of them.

5. Turn around and spray again with the oil.

6. Place the anchovies in the basket of the Air fryer so that they are not on top of each other.

7. We select 180ºC, 15 minutes.

8. Do the same per batch until you have all the fried anchovies.

Nutritional Information

- Calories: 69
- Carbohydrates: 4.4g
- Fat: 3.8g
- Protein: 4.2g
- Sugar: 0g
- Cholesterol: 26mg

Banana Bread

• Servings:1• Preparation time: 10 minutes• Cook time: 40 minutes •

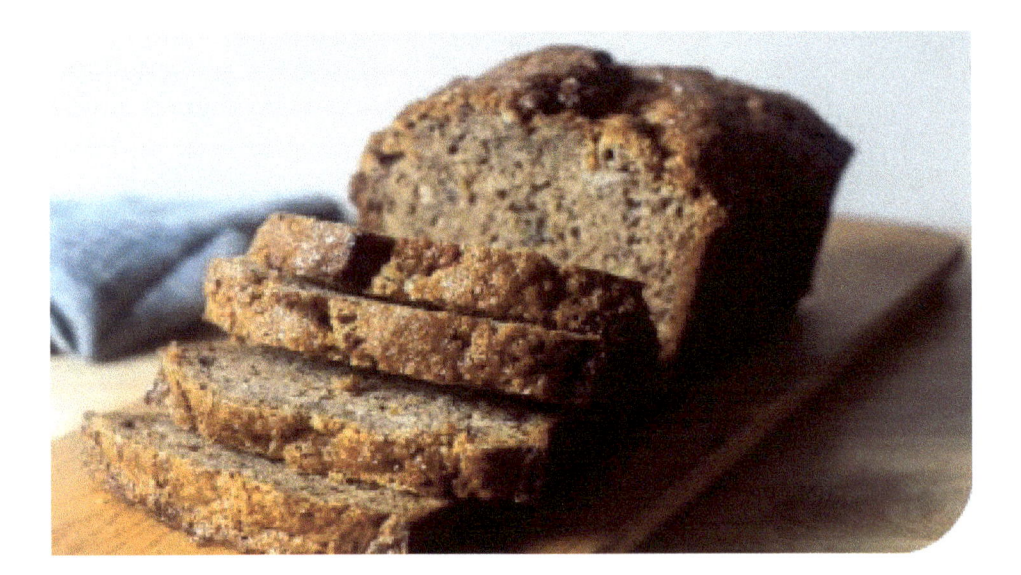

FUITY

Ingredients

- 1 oz. unsalted butter, softened
- 3 ½ oz. of sugar
- 1 egg, beaten
- 2 ripe bananas pureed
- ½ tsp of pure vanilla extract
- ½ oz. all-purpose flour
- ½ tsp of baking soda
- 1/3 tsp of salt
- 1 ½ oz. of chopped walnuts
- Non-stick spray oil

Steps to Cook

1. Mix the butter with the sugar.

2. Mix the eggs, banana puree, and vanilla. Set aside.

3. Select Preheat, in the air fryer adjust the temperature to 150°C.

4. Sift the flour, baking soda, and salt.

5. Blend the dry ingredients into the wet ingredients until combined. Then mix the chopped nuts.

6. Grease 1 mini-loaf pan with cooking spray and fill it with the mixture. Place in preheated air fryer.

7. Select Desserts, set to 40 minutes.

Nutritional Information

- Calories: 247
- Carbohydrates: 39g
- Fat: 8.8g
- Protein: 3.8g
- Sugar: 19g
- Cholesterol: 51mg

Salad With Cod Fritter Balls

• Servings: 4 • Preparation time: 5 minutes • Cook time: 20 minutes •

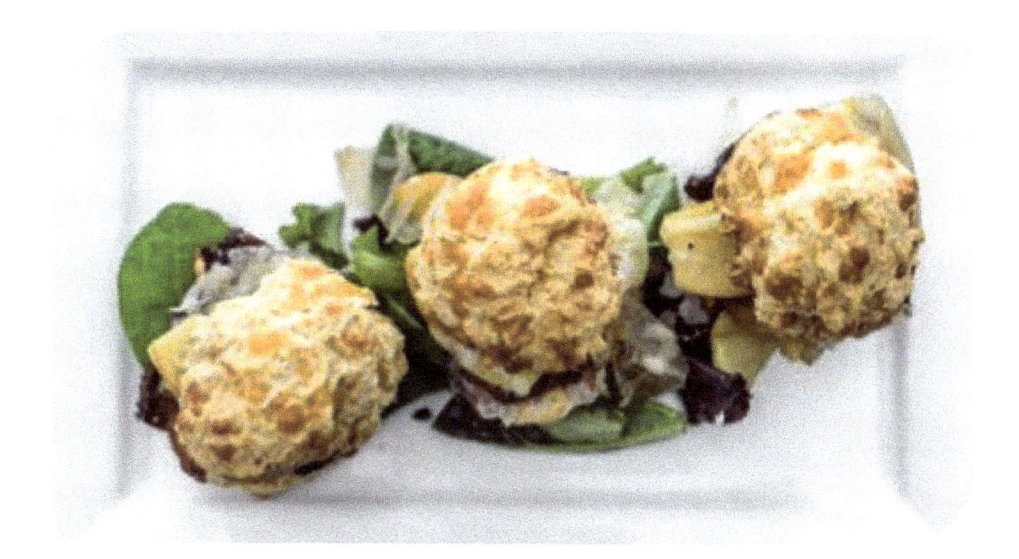

Ingredients

- 1 romaine lettuce
- 1 pot of Cesar sauce, or homemade Cesar sauce
- 1 bag of mini cod fritters
- Oil
- Salt

Steps to Cook

1. We put the fritters in the Air fryer for 15 minutes at 180ºC, pulverized with a little oil.

2. Chop the lettuce and place in a salad bowl.

3. Put a little salt on the lettuce and place the fritters on it, well distributed.

4. Add the Cesar sauce.

Nutritional Information

- Calories: 127
- Carbohydrates: 7.8g
- Fat: 6.61g
- Protein: 8.6g
- Sugar: 0.54g
- Cholesterol: 35mg

Air Fryer Cookbook

Battered Of Fish

• Servings: 4 • Preparation time: 5 minutes • Cook time: 15 minutes •

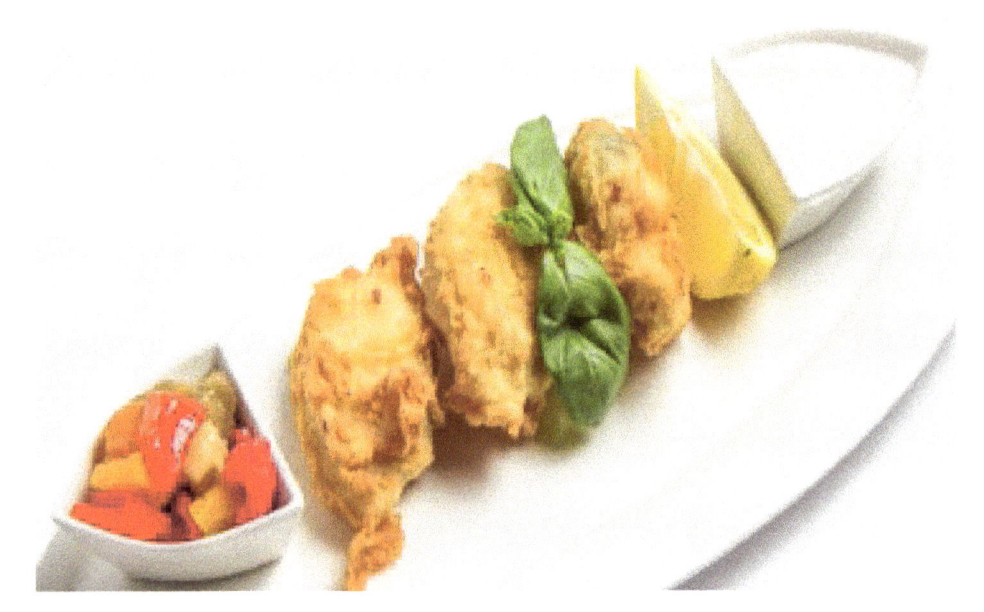

AMAZINGLY DELICIOUS

Ingredients

- 8 fillets of hake
- 2 eggs
- Flour
- Salt
- Extra virgin olive oil

Steps to Cook

1. Put the eggs on a plate and beat very well.

2. Add the flour little by little while continuing to stir until obtaining a dense cream.

3. Put salt on the fish fillets.

4. Submerge well in the dense cream that you have prepared and now you only have to transfer the fish to the air fryer preheated with a few threads of oil on top.

5. Select 200°C for 15 minutes.

Nutritional Information

- Calories: 69
- Carbohydrates: 4.4g
- Fat: 3.8g
- Protein: 4.2g
- Sugar: 0g
- Cholesterol: 26mg

Chapter 6

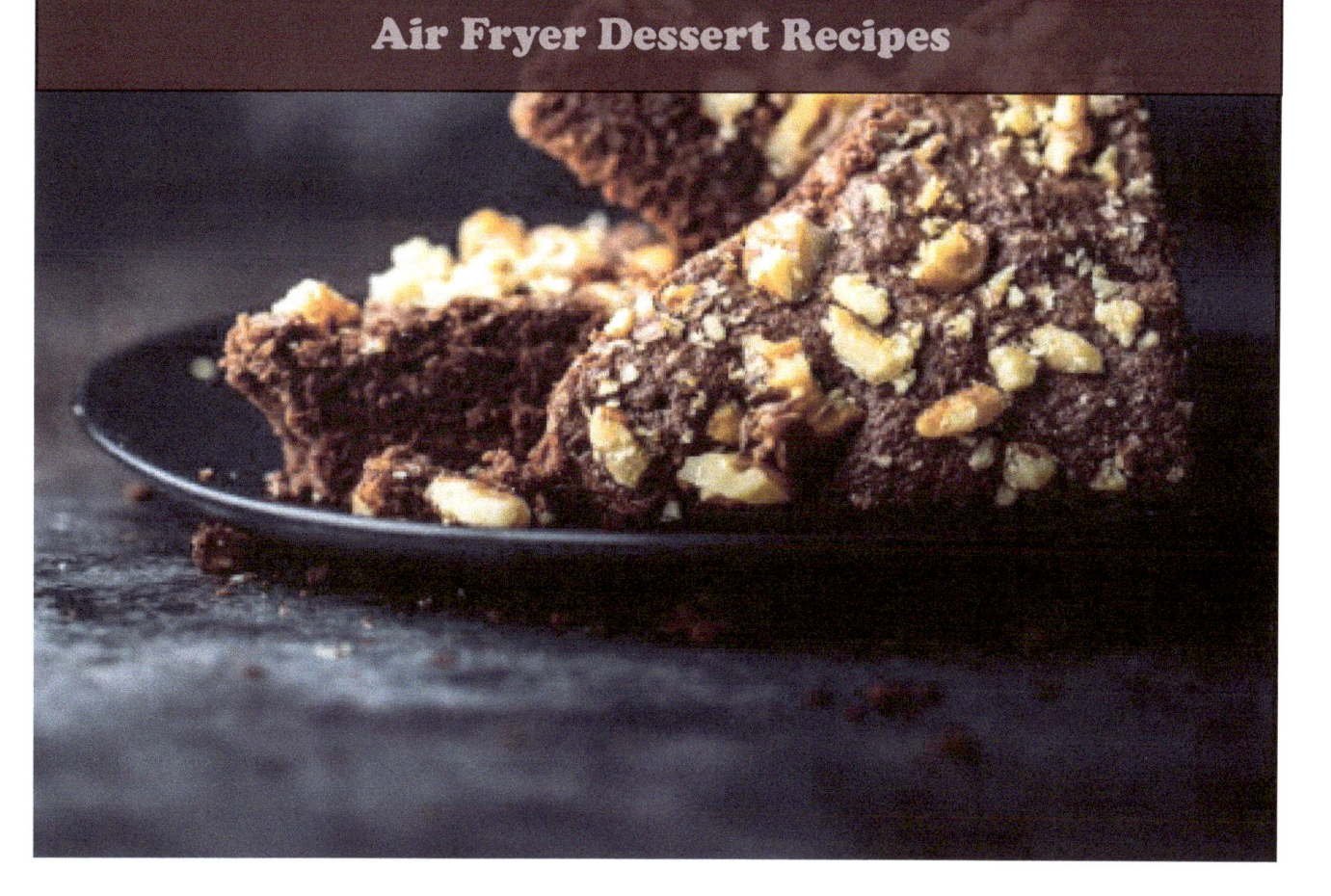

Air Fryer Dessert Recipes

Air Fryer Cookbook

Chocolate Muffins

• Servings: 6 • Preparation time: 10 minutes • Cook time: 15 minutes •

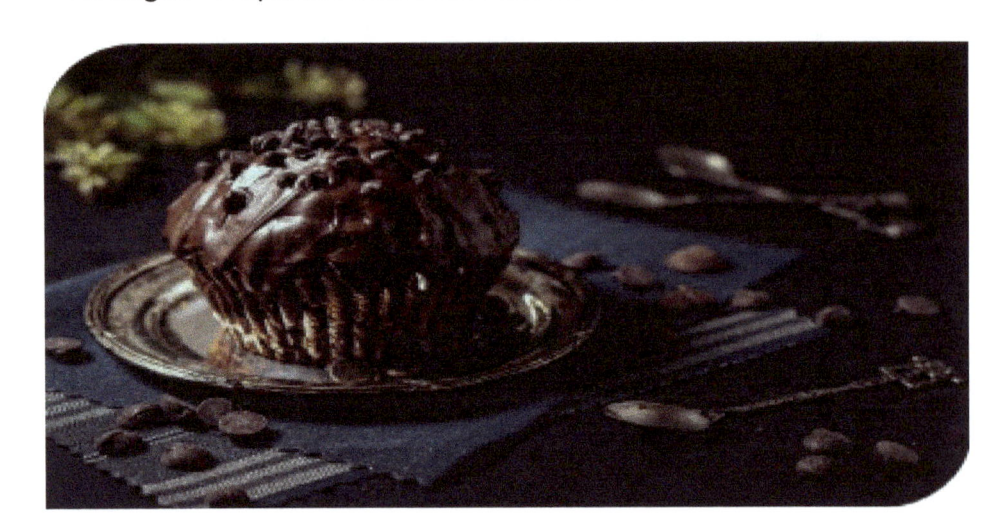

CHOCOLATY

Ingredients

- 1 ½ oz. granulated sugar
- ½ cup coconut milk or soy milk
- 1/3 cup coconut oil, liquid
- 1 tsp of vanilla extract
- 4 oz. all-purpose flour
- 3 tsp cocoa powder
- 1 tsp baking powder
- ½ tsp of baking soda
- a pinch of salt
- 3 oz. of chocolate chips
- 1 oz. pistachios, cracked (Optional)
- Non-stick spray oil

Steps to Cook

1. Put the sugar, coconut milk, coconut oil, and vanilla extract in a small bowl. Set aside.

2. Mix the flour, cocoa powder, baking powder, baking soda, and salt in a separate bowl and set aside.

3. Mix the dry ingredients with the wet ingredients gradually, until smooth. Then mix with the chocolate and pistachio.

4. Select Preheat, in the air fryer adjust the temperature to 150°C.

5. Grease the muffin tins with cooking spray and pour the mixture until they are full to ¾.

6. Carefully place the muffin tins in the preheated air fryer. Select Desserts, set the time to 15 minutes.

7. Remove the muffins when the cooking is done and let them cool for 10 minutes before serving.

Nutritional Information

- Calories: 690
- Carbohydrates: 79.2g
- Fat: 38g
- Protein: 9.9g
- Sugar: 15g
- Cholesterol: 125mg

SPONGY

Sweet Sponge Cake

• Servings: 10 • Preparation time: 10 minutes • Cook time: 50 minutes •

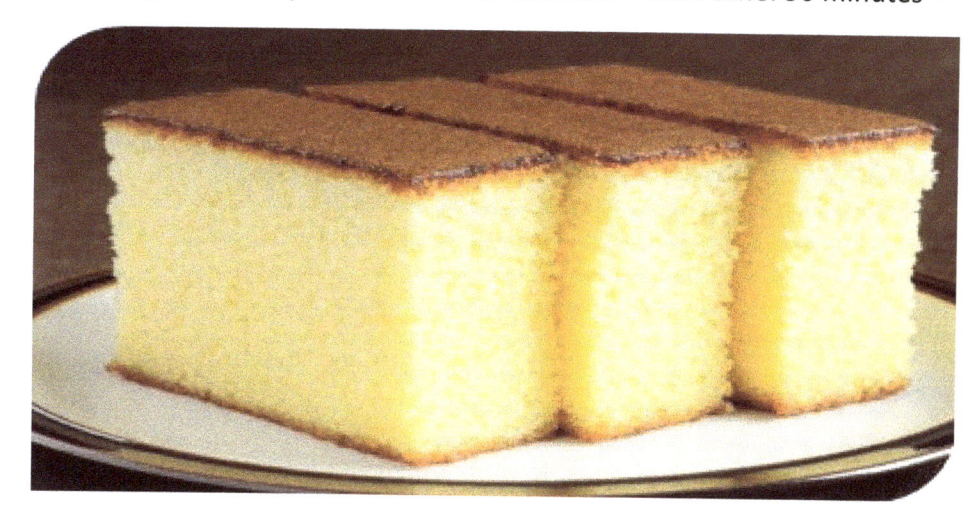

Ingredients

- ½ lb flour for
- yeast pastry
- ½ lb of sugar
- 3 medium eggs
- 3 tbsp olive oil
- Orange zest
- ¾ lb chopped pistachio
- 1 envelope of yeast

Steps to Cook

1. Separate the yolks from the eggs. Mount the egg whites until stiff with the mixer and gradually incorporate the sugar.

2. Mix until you get a thick white cream.

3. Separately, beat the yolks with the oil and the orange zest. Incorporate this mixture with the whites, mix in an enveloping way and finally incorporate the flour and yeast with a sieve. When everything is well mixed, add the pistachios. You can use a circular mold greased with oil and flour or kitchen paper that is more comfortable. Add the cake batter to the pan.

4. Preheat the Air fryer for a few minutes at 1600C. Put the mold in the basket of the Air fryer and program the timer for about 30 minutes at 1600C temperature.

5. While it is cooking prepare the lemon cream.

6. To do this, gradually mix the white with the sugar, add the lemon juice and add the sour cream and mix until obtaining a thick cream and ready.

Nutritional Information

- Calories: 110
- Carbohydrates: 23g
- Fat: 1g
- Protein: 2.1g
- Sugar: 14g
- Cholesterol: 39mg

Egg Custard

SWEET

• Servings: 4 • Preparation time: 10 minutes • Cook time: 60 minutes •

Ingredients

- 1 ¼ cup milk
- 3 eggs
- 3 oz. of sugar

Steps to Cook

1. Put the sugar in a saucepan, reserving two tablespoons for later. Add a little water. With very low heat melt the sugar until it is all liquid and caramelized.

2. Immediately pour into the pudding molds. It is important to do it right away because the caramel solidifies very quickly on cooling.

3. In a separate bowl, beat the eggs with the help of some rods. When they start frothing, add the milk and mix everything very well.

4. Once the mixture is homogeneous, pour into the molds to which you will have previously put the caramel.

5. Then preheat the Air fryer for a few minutes to 160ºC.

6. Then cook the custards in a bain-marie in the Air fryer. To do this, arrange the custards inside the basket of the Air fryer in a container with water ensuring that the water reaches half of the containers but ensuring that no water enters them.

7. Put the container with the flan and the medium water bathing them in the Air fryer and cook everything at medium temperature 160ºC for about 1 hour.

8. To check if the flans are cooked, shake gently and if they have the consistent appearance of the flans when they are moved, they are ready. Otherwise, if they look very liquid, bake them in a bain-marie a little more.

Nutritional Information

- Calories: 146.6
- Carbohydrates: 15.5g
- Fat: 6.5g
- Protein: 7.1g
- Sugar: 15.5g
- Cholesterol: 118.4mg

Roasted Apples

• Servings: 4 • Preparation time: 2 minutes • Cook time: 20 minutes •

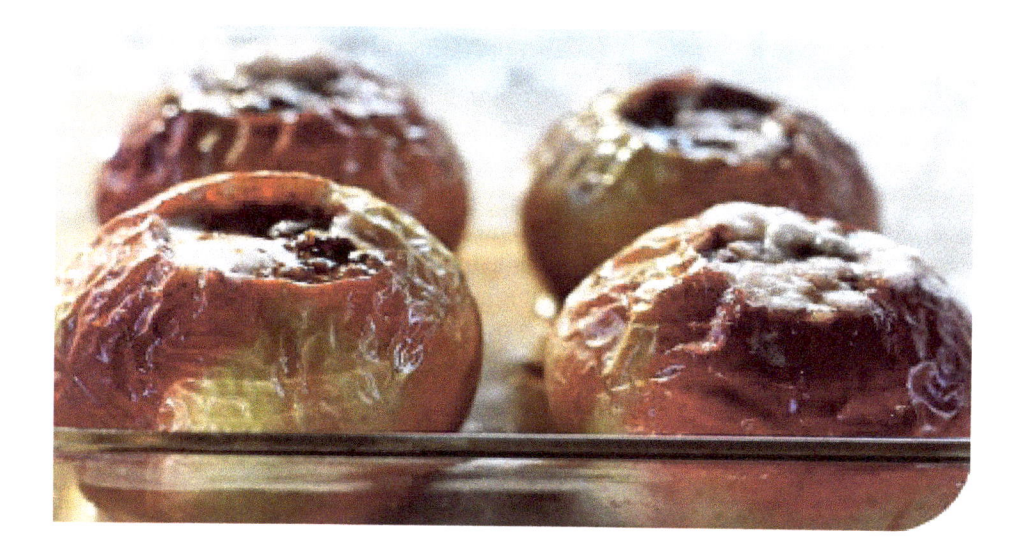

HEALTHY

Ingredients

- 4 apples
- 4 teaspoons of butter
- 4 teaspoons of honey
- A little cinnamon powder

Steps to Cook

1. Discourage apples.

2. Incorporate, in the center of each apple, a teaspoon of butter, another of honey and a little cinnamon.

3. Preheat the Air fryer for a few minutes at 180ºC.

4. Put the apples in the basket of the Air fryer and set the timer for 20 minutes at 180ºC.

Nutritional Information

- Calories: 98
- Carbohydrates: 14g
- Fat: 7g
- Protein: 0g
- Sugar: 10g
- Cholesterol: 300mg

Air Fryer Cookbook

Homemade Muffins

• Servings:6• Preparation time:5 minutes• Cook time: 20 minutes •

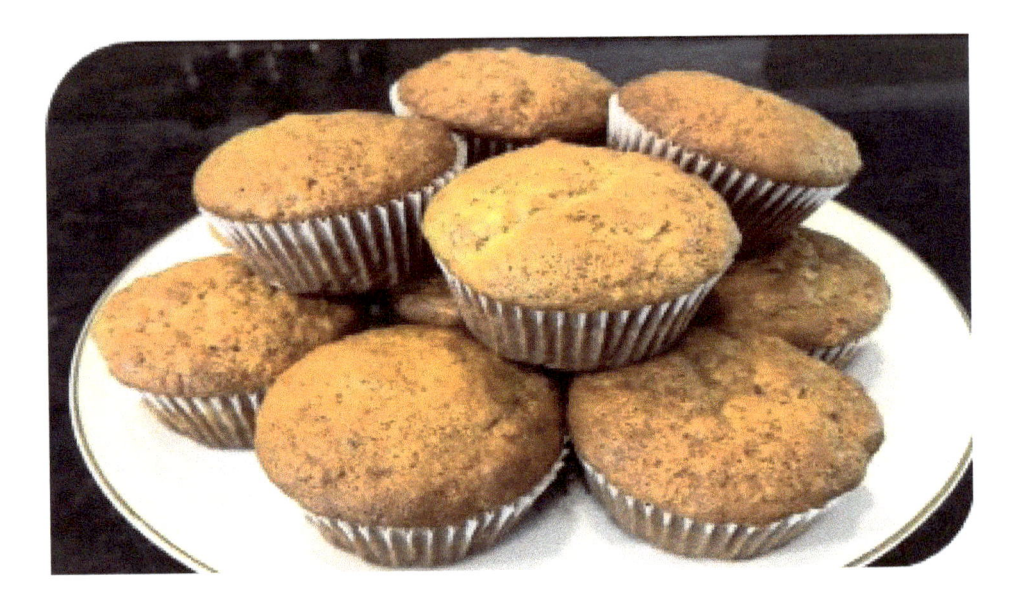

SWEET

Ingredients

- 6 tbsp of olive oil
- 3 ½ oz. of sugar
- 2 eggs
- 3 ½ oz. of flour
- 1 tsp of baking powder Royal
- Lemon zest

Steps to Cook

1. Beat the eggs with the sugar, with the help of a whisk. Add the oil little by little, without stopping stirring, until you get a soft and fluffy cream.

2. Then add the lemon zest.

3. Finally, incorporate the sifted flour with the yeast into the previous mixture and mix in an enveloping way.

4. Fill the 2/3 parts of the muffin cups with the dough.

5. Preheat the Air fryer a few minutes to 180ºC and when it is ready to put the molds in the basket.

6. Set the timer for about 20 minutes at a temperature of 180ºC, until golden brown

Nutritional Information

- Calories: 168.7
- Carbohydrates:23.6g
- Fat: 6.5g
- Protein: 3.9g
- Sugar: 14g
- Cholesterol: 22.2mg

Blueberry And Orange Cake

• Servings: 6 • Preparation time: 10 minutes • Cook time: 15 minutes •

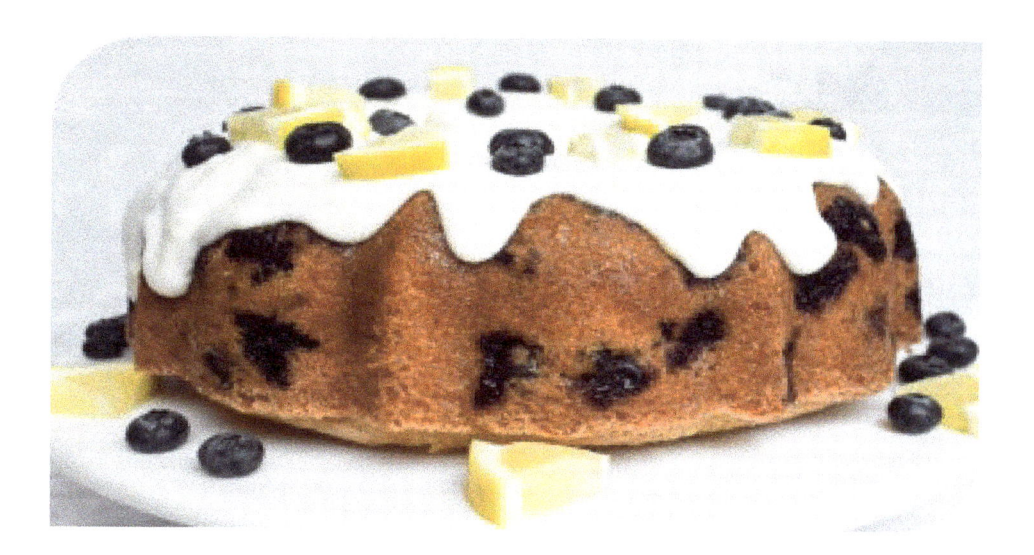

YUMMY
___

Ingredients

- 4 ¼ oz. all-purpose flour
- 2 1/3 oz. of sugar
- 4 g baking powder
- 1 tsp of baking soda
- Pinch salt
- 3 ½ oz. blueberries
- 1 egg
- 1/3 cup orange juice
- ¼ cup of vegetable oil
- 1 orange, zest
- Non-stick spray oil Salt

Steps to Cook

1. Combine flour, baking powder, baking soda, salt, and blueberries in large bowl.

2. Whisk together the egg, orange juice, oil, and orange zest in a separate bowl.

3. Mix the wet and dry ingredients until well combined.

4. Grease the muffin tins with cooking spray and pour the mixture until they are full to ¾.

5. Select Preheat, in the air fryer adjust the temperature to 150°C.

6. Carefully place the muffin tins in the preheated air fryer. You may need to work in parts.

7. Select Desserts, set the time to 15 minutes.

Nutritional Information

- Calories: 493
- Carbohydrates: 66g
- Fat: 25g
- Protein: 4g
- Sugar: 14g
- Cholesterol: 98mg

Palm Trees Hojaldre

• Servings: 4 • Preparation time: 5 minutes • Cook time: 10 minutes •

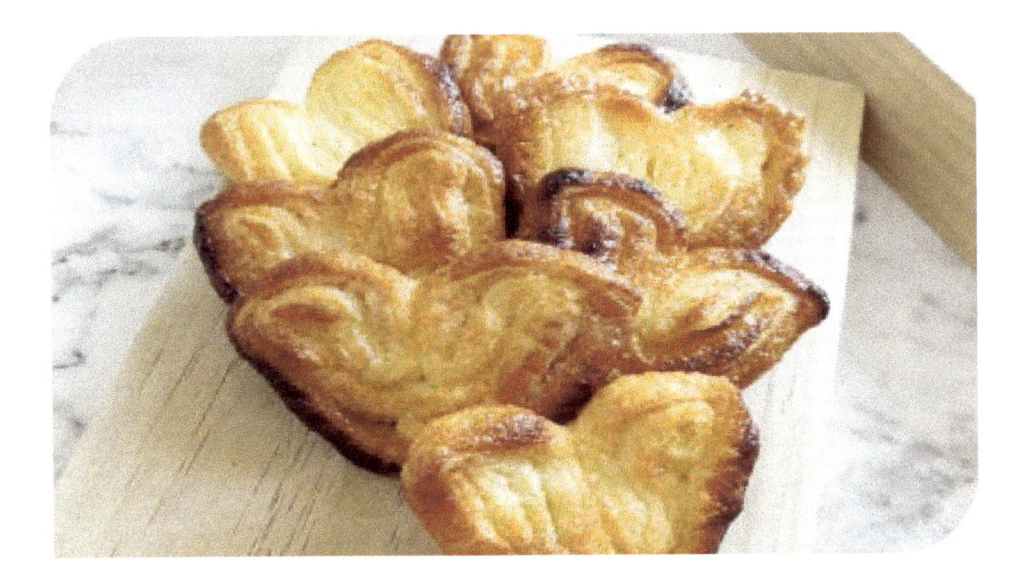

FRUITY

Ingredients

- 1 sheet of puff pastry
- Sugar

Steps to Cook

1. Roll out the puff pastry sheet.

2. Pour the sugar on top and fold the puff pastry sheet in half.

3. Put a thin layer of sugar on top again and fold the dough again puff pastry in half.

4. Roll up the puff pastry sheet from both ends towards the center (creating the shape of the palm tree).

5. Cut into sheets 5-8 mm thick.

6. Preheat the Air fryer to 180°C and put the palm trees in the basket.

7. Set the timer about 10 minutes to 180°C.

Nutritional Information

- Calories: 120
- Carbohydrates: 10g
- Fat: 8g
- Protein: 4g
- Sugar: 10g
- Cholesterol: 300mg

Coconut Balls

• Servings: 6 • Preparation time: 10 minutes • Cook time: 15 minutes •

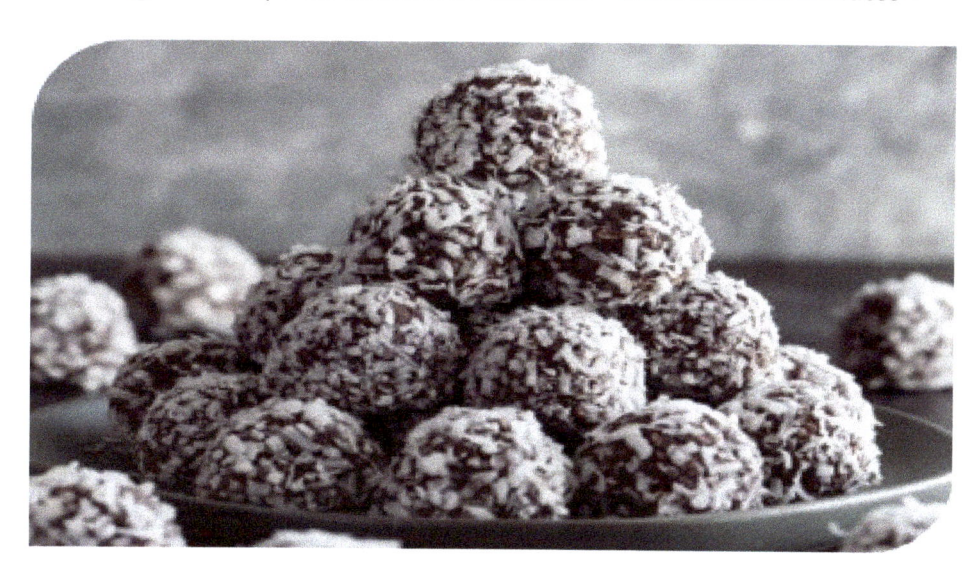

LOW FAT

Ingredients

- 3 ½ oz of sweetened condensed milk
- 1 egg white
- ½ tsp almond extract
- ½ tsp of vanilla extract
- a pinch of salt
- 6 oz. unsweetened and crumbled coconut

Steps to Cook

1. Mix the condensed milk, the egg white, the almond extract and the salt in a bowl. Add 5 oz. of grated coconut and mix until well combined. The mixture must be able to maintain its shape.

2. Shape 38mm balls with your hands. On a separate plate, add 1 oz. of grated coconut.

3. Roll the coconut macaroons into the grated coconut until covered.

4. Select Preheat, in the air fryer adjust the temperature to 150°C. Add the coconut macaroons to the preheated air fryer.

5. Select Desserts, set the time to 15 minutes.

6. Let the macaroni cool for 5-10 minutes and serve when they finish cooling.

Nutritional Information

- Calories: 97.5
- Carbohydrates: 8.5g
- Fat: 6.7g
- Protein: 1.2g
- Sugar: 2.6g
- Cholesterol: 0.1mg

Air Fryer Cookbook

Cheddar Cheese Bites

• Servings: 8 • Preparation time: 1 minutes • Cook time: 20 minutes •

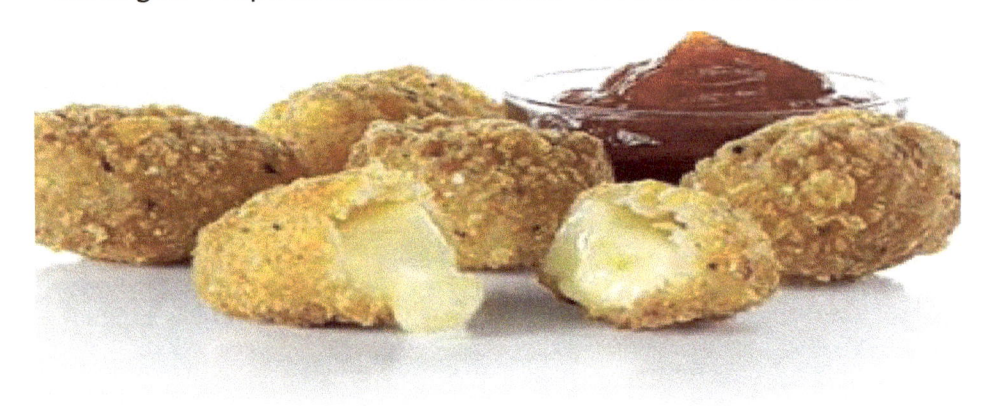

JUICY

Ingredients

- 1 8 squares of cheddar cheese
- Mashed potatoes
- Flour
- Egg and breadcrumbs
- Extra virgin olive oil

Steps to Cook

1. Make the mashed potatoes as you like.

2. Cut the cheddar cheese into small squares.

3. Take a piece of cheese and wrap it with a thin layer of mashed potatoes.

4. When you have the 8 pieces wrapped in the mashed potatoes, take it to the freezer for about 30 minutes.

5. Go through flour and shake.

6. Go through the beaten egg, breadcrumbs, again through the beaten egg and again through the breadcrumbs.

7. Take to the refrigerator at least 30 minutes.

8. Place in the basket of the Air fryer and paint well with extra virgin olive oil.

9. Select 20 minutes, 180ºC.

Nutritional Information

- Calories: 130
- Carbohydrates: 20g
- Fat: 3.5g
- Protein: 3g
- Sugar: 1g
- Cholesterol: 300mg

Mini Potato and Egg Pizza

• Servings: 6-8 • Preparation time: 10 minutes • Cook time: 35minutes •

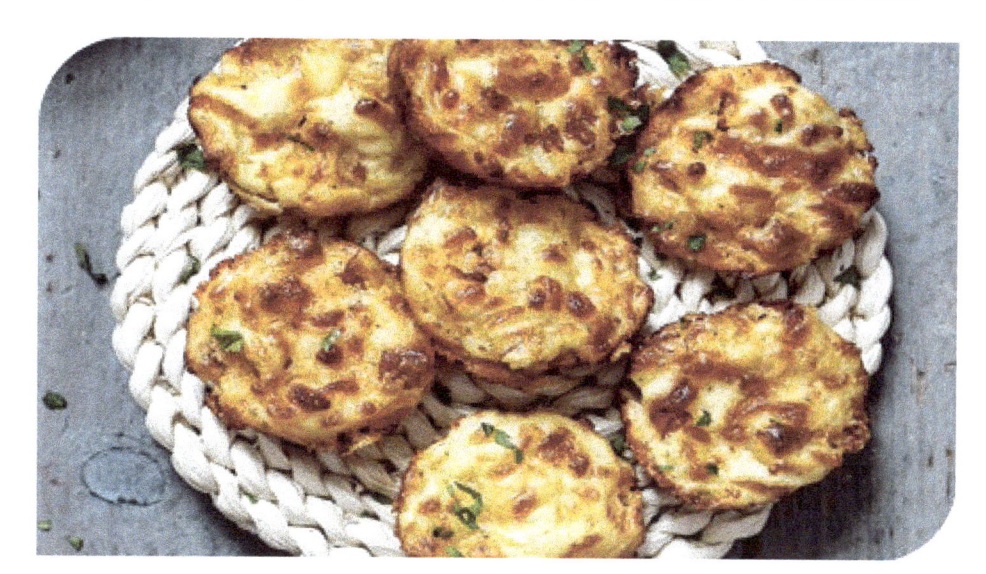

PALATABLE

Ingredients

- ½ lb of wheat flour
- ¼ lb of water
- 5 tsp of extra virgin olive oil
- 2 tsp of salt
- 2 tsp of yeast
- 8 eggs
- 2 potatoes
- extra virgin olive oil
- Salt
- Ketchup
- Oregano
- Bacon
- Grated cheese

Steps to Cook

1. Peel the potatoes and cut them into a long, thick stick. Put salt, a little oil and mix.

2. Put them in the pan of the Air fryer and select 30 minutes. Reserve.

3. Continue with the pizza dough. For this, put in the in the food processor with kneading hook, the flour, water, oil, salt and yeast. Knead at low speed for at least 5 minutes. Make a ball and let it rest for 30 minutes. Divide the dumpling into 8 equal parts.

4. We spread the masses. Put a small layer of tomato sauce and sprinkle with oregano. Place the potatoes on the edge of the pizza dough. Press a little so that they are well fixed in the dough. Take to the preheated air fryer, 180ºC, 15 minutes.

5. Remove the mini pizza slices and add a layer of chopped bacon and on the bacon crack an egg in each mini pizza. Cover with grated cheese on the part of the white, leaving the yolk in sight. Return to the air fryer, 180ºC, another 10 to 20 minutes

Nutritional Information

- Calories: 179.7
- Carbohydrates: 34.2g
- Fat: 3.3g
- Protein: 5.2g
- Sugar: 0.6g
- Cholesterol: 0mg

Air Fryer Cookbook

Chocolate and walnut cake

• Servings: 2-4 • Preparation time: 5 minutes • Cook time: 20 minutes •

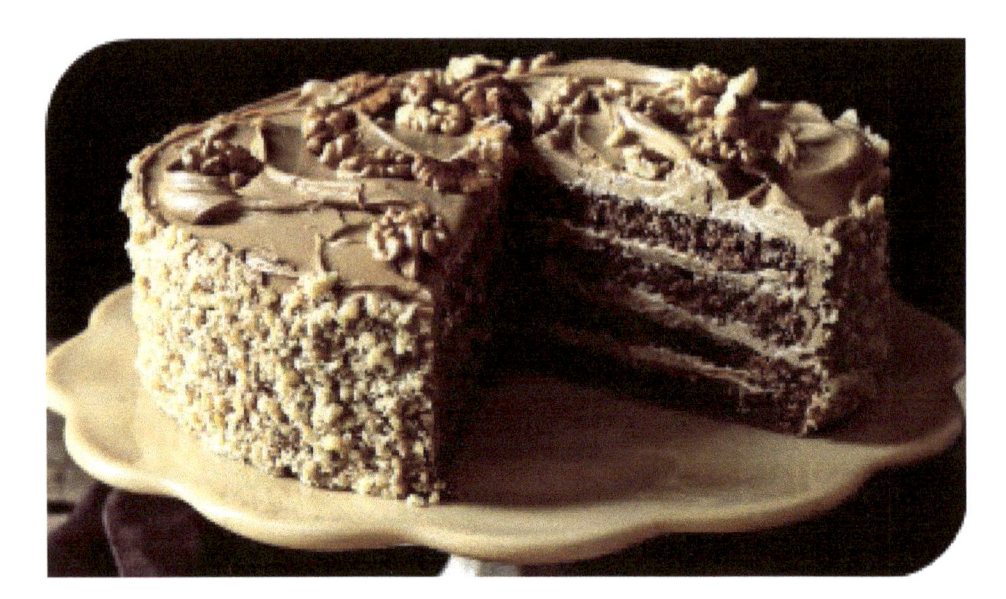

CHOCOLATE FLAVOR

Ingredients

- 2 ¼ oz dark chocolate
- 2 butter spoons
- 1 egg
- 3 spoonfuls of sugar
- 2 oz. flour
- 1 envelope Royal yeast
- Chopped walnuts

Steps to Cook

1. Melt the dark chocolate with the butter over low heat. Once melted, put in a bowl.

2. Incorporate the egg, sugar, flour, yeast and finally the chopped nuts.

3. Beat well by hand until uniform dough is obtained.

4. Put the dough in a silicone mold or oven suitable for incorporation in the basket of the Air fryer.

5. Preheat the Air fryer for a few minutes at 1800C.

6. Set the timer for 20 minutes at 1800C and when it has cooled, remove from the mold.

Nutritional Information

- Calories: 310
- Carbohydrates: 44g
- Fat: 14g
- Protein: 5g
- Sugar: 27g
- Cholesterol: 70mg

Light Cheese Cake

• Servings: 8 • Preparation time: 5 minutes • Cook time: 55 minutes •

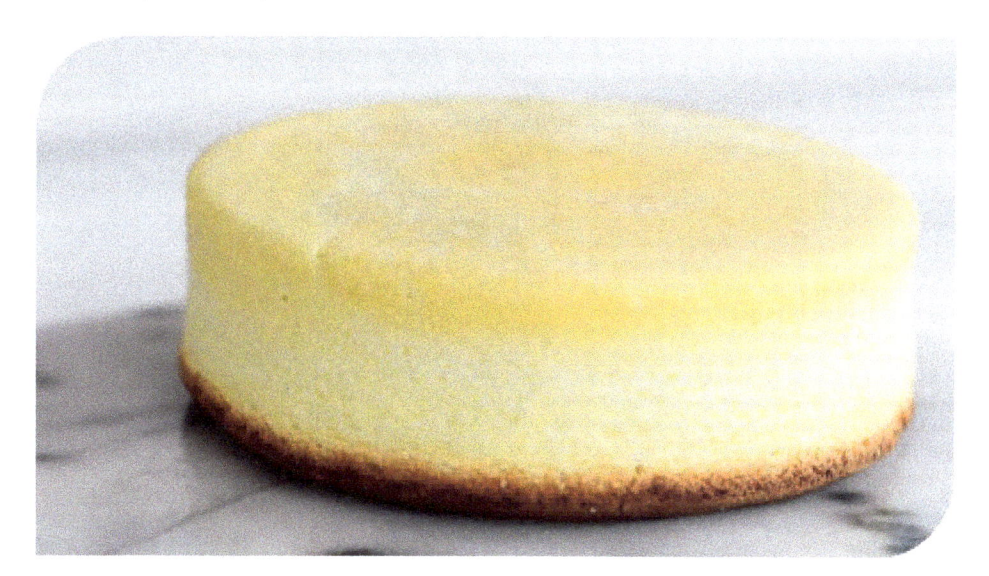

SPONGY

Ingredients

- 1 lb of cottage cheese
- 3 whole eggs
- 2 tbsp of sweetener powder
- 2 tbsp of oat bran
- ½ tbsp of baking yeast
- 2 tbsp of cinnamon
- 2 tbsp vanilla flavoring
- 1 lemon (the skin)

Steps to Cook

1. Mix the cottage cheese, the sweetener, the cinnamon, the vanilla flavor and the lemon zest in a bowl. Mix very well until you get a homogeneous cream.

2. Incorporate the eggs one by one.

3. Finally, add the oats and yeast, mixing well.

4. Put all the mixture in a container so that it fits in the Air fryer.

5. Preheat the Air fryer for a few minutes at 180°C.

6. Put the mold in the basket of the Air fryer and adjust the timer for about 20 minutes at 180°C.

Nutritional Information

- Calories: 222
- Carbohydrates: 9g
- Fat: 14g
- Protein: 18g
- Sugar: 7g
- Cholesterol: 160mg

Blackberry Pie With Cheese

• Servings: 4 • Preparation time: 5 minutes • Cook time: 20-30 minutes •

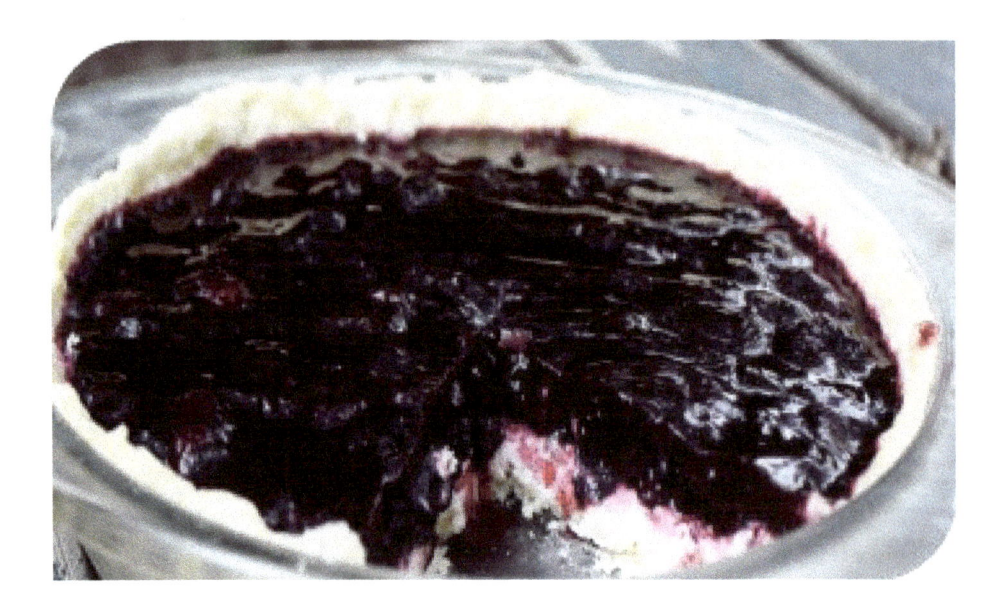

DELICIOUS

Ingredients

• 2 cups blackberry

• 1 cup of sugar

• 1 tbsp of lemon juice

• enough flour to spread

• ½ lb of puff pastry

• ½ cups cream cheese, diced

• enough egg, to varnish

• enough of icing sugar, to decorate

Steps to Cook

1. Preheat the air fryer to 200°C.

2. In a saucepan cook the blackberries with the sugar for about 30 minutes over low heat or until it has a thick consistency, add the lemon juice and mix well. Let cool and reserve.

3. On a floured surface spread the puff pastry approximately 3 mm thick and with the help of a 10 cm diameter round cutter cut discs.

4. Fill the puff pastry discs with the blackberry jam and cream cheese, close and with the help of your hands make a fold, place on a tray and varnish with egg.

5. Put in the air fryer for 20 minutes or until golden, let cool and decorate with icing sugar.

Nutritional Information

• Calories: 470

• Carbohydrates: 57 g

• Fat: 27g

• Protein: 6g

• Sugar: 33g

• Cholesterol: 220mg

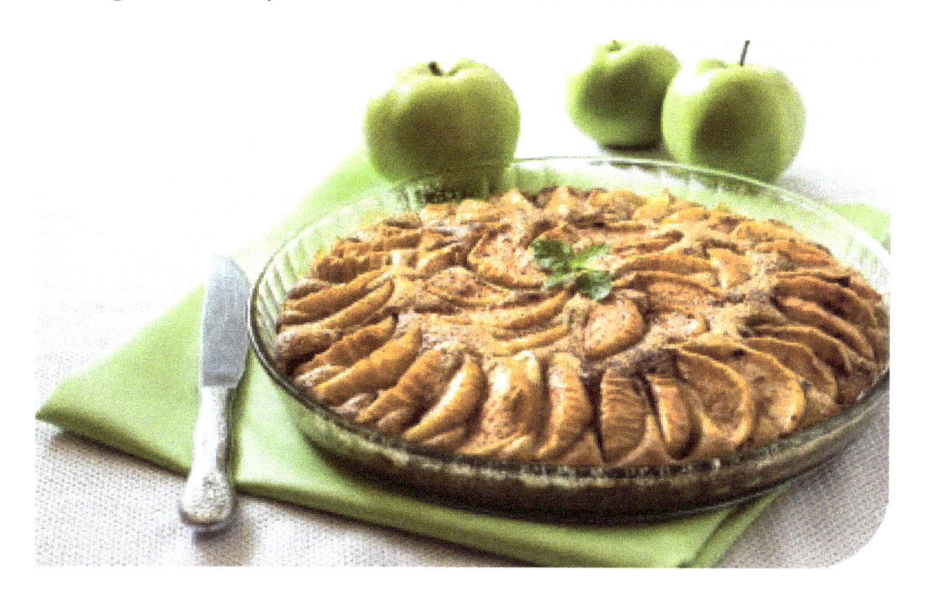

HEALTHY

Apple Pie and Sweet Milk

• Servings: 6-8 • Preparation time: 5 minutes • Cook time: 20 minutes •

Ingredients

- 3 apples
- 1/3 cups cranberry
- ½ cups of walnut
- ½ cups of rum
- enough flour to spread
- ½ lb of puff pastry
- ¾ cups of sweet milk
- 1 egg, to varnish
- enough walnut, finely chopped, to decorate

Steps to Cook

1. Preheat the air fryer to 200°C.

2. For the filling, peel and cut the apples into very thin sheets, place in a bowl and mix with the walnuts, blueberries and rum. Macerate for 30 minutes, drain very well and reserve.

3. Spread the puff pastry on a floured surface 3 mm thick, with the help of a 10 cm diameter cutter that cuts discs.

4. Fill the puff pastry discs with the apples and a little sweet milk, with the help of your hands make folds to close the empanadas. Place on a tray, varnish with egg and sprinkle with walnuts.

5. Put in the air fryer for 20 minutes or until golden. Serve with milk or coffee.

Nutritional Information

- Calories: 750
- Carbohydrates: 82g
- Fat: 37g
- Protein: 15g
- Sugar: 66g
- Cholesterol: 155mg

Lemon Cake

• Servings:6• Preparation time: 5 minutes• Cook time: 30 minutes •

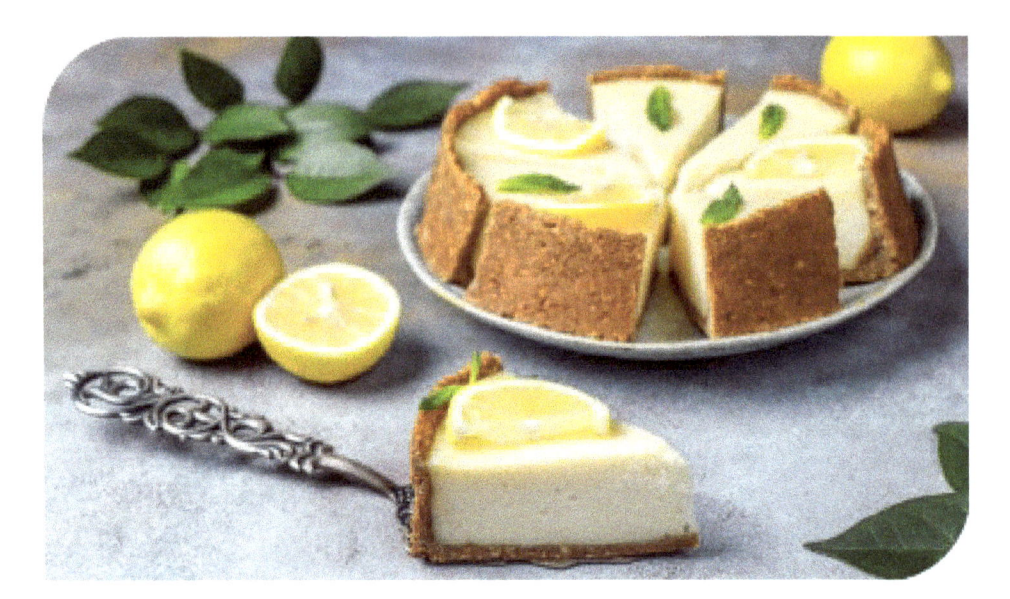

LEMONADE

Ingredients

- ¼ lb all-purpose flour
- 1 tsp baking powder
- a pinch of salt
- 3 oz. unsalted butter, softened
- ¼ lb granulated sugar
- 1 large egg
- ½ oz. of fresh lemon juice
- 1 lemon, lemon zest
- 2 oz. of whey

Steps to Cook

1. Mix the flour, baking powder, and salt in a bowl. Set aside. Add the softened butter to an electric mixer and beat until smooth and fluffy. Approximately 3 minutes. Beat the sugar in the butter for 1 minute.

2. Whisk the flour mixture in the butter until completely united, for about 1 minute. Add the egg, lemon juice, and lemon zest. Mix until everything is completely united. Slowly pour in the buttermilk while mixing on medium speed.

3. Add the mixture to a greased mini-loaf pan on top.

4. Select Preheat, in the air fryer adjust the temperature to 160°C. Place the cake in the preheated air fryer. Select Pan, set the time to 30 minutes.

Nutritional Information

- Calories: 326
- Carbohydrates: 12.1g
- Fat: 25.2g
- Protein: 13.4g
- Sugar: 0.5g
- Cholesterol: 10mg

Healthy Carrot Chips

• Servings:3 • Preparation time: 5 minutes • Cook time: 20-25 minutes •

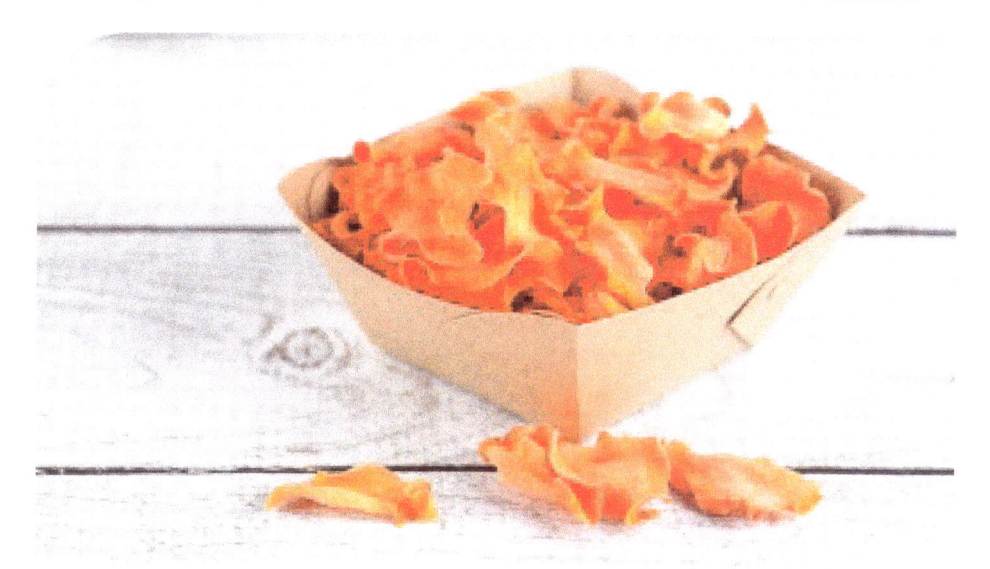

HEALTHY

Ingredients

• carrots to taste

• 2 tablespoons extra virgin olive oil

• salt to taste

Steps to Cook

1. Wash the carrots very well and remove the ends.

2. Cut the carrots into very thin slices, either using a mandolin or with a food processor.

3. Add the oil and with clean hands, spread it over all the carrots. Put the carrot slices in the basket of your air fryer and program it at 165ºC for 20-25 minutes, depending on the amount of carrots you make.

4. Every 5-7 minutes open the basket and shake it vigorously so that they are removed, and put the basket back inside so that they continue to be made. Watch from the 15th minute that they do not burn, since it depends on the amount you do can be done before. Take out the carrots, put some salt on them and ready.

Nutritional Information

• Calories: 35

• Carbohydrates: 8g

• Fat: 2g

• Protein: 1g

• Sugar: 5g

• Cholesterol: 300mg

Focaccia

• Servings:4• Preparation time: 45 minutes• Cook time: 20 minutes •

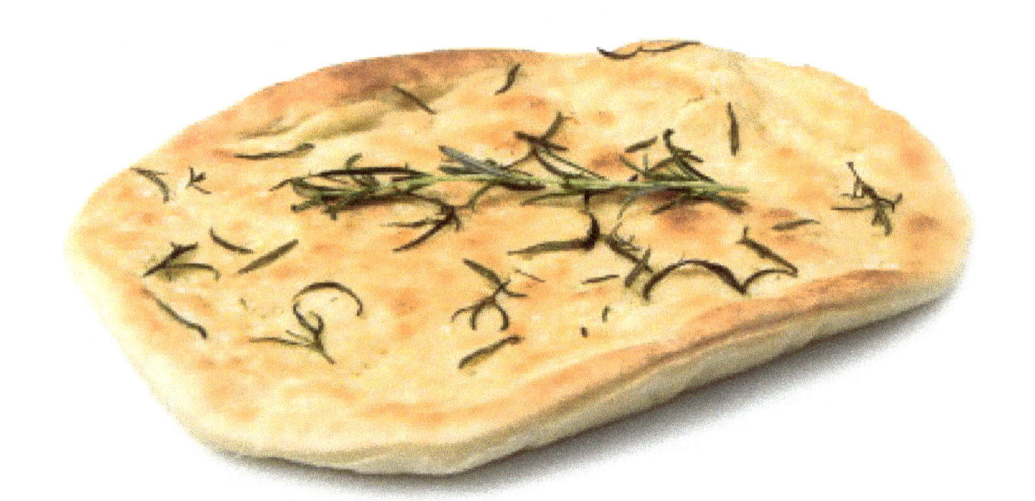

PALATABLE

Ingredients

- ½ oz. dry yeast
- ½ cup warm water
- 1 cup baker's flour
- Mass
- ½ oz. dry yeast
- ½ pound baker's flour
- Warm water with Nec

Steps to Cook

1. Assemble the sponge for 40 minutes. Assemble the dough, unite with the sponge for 45 minutes, knead degassing until the dough joins and becomes smooth.

2. Assemble the pastries, they can roll 20-gram loaves, or in a source place the extended dough, let it take half an hour, in the extended dough they can drip olive oil, rosemary, tomatoes, onion into slices and bake at 180ºC 10 minutes approximately both bread and focaccia.

Nutritional Information

- Calories: 387.9
- Carbohydrates: 64.4g
- Fat: 9.9g
- Protein: 9g
- Sugar: 0.2g
- Cholesterol: 0mg

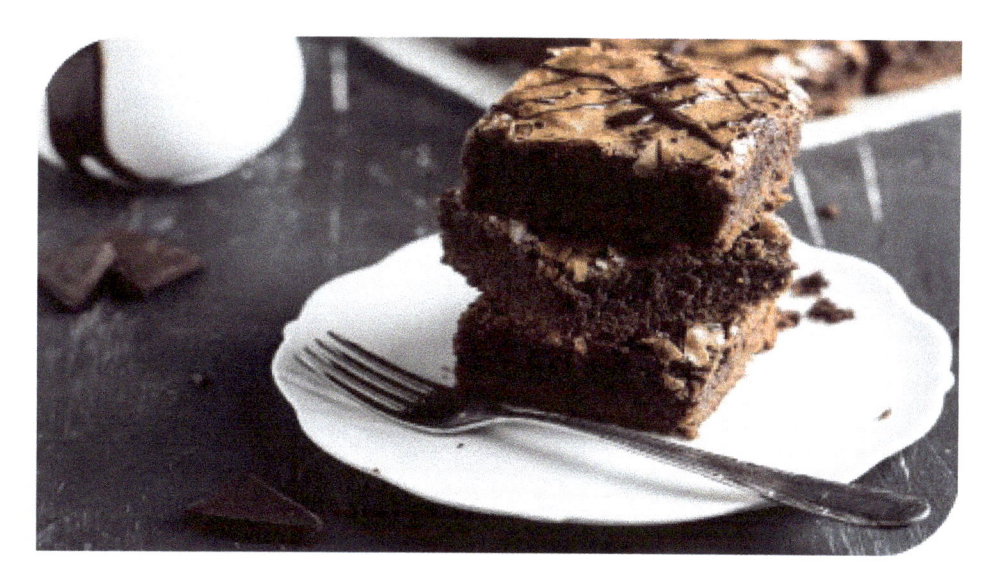

DELICIOUS

Ingredients

• 2 eggs

• 1 homemade chocolate soy yogurt

• 1 container of yogurt sugar

• 2 containers of sponge cake flour

• ½ container of oil

• ½ sachet baking powder

• Orange zest

Chocolate cake

• Servings: 2 • Preparation time: 5 minutes • Cook time: 40 minutes •

Steps to Cook

1. Preheat deep fryer 175°C 5 minutes

2. In a bowl put the eggs, the yogurt and sugar, beat and then add the flour, the yeast, the oil and the orange zest.

3. Mix all.

4. In the bucket of the fryer (mold on purpose for the fryer) but also a mold that burns inside. Put the oven paper down the mold and add the dough.

5. Put in a fryer Cupcakes program 15 minutes at 150°C. Then make some cross cuts on the cake and put another 15 minutes with the same temperature. If it is not cooked inside, add about 5 minutes more at 140°C.

Nutritional Information

• Calories: 424

• Carbohydrates: 58g

• Fat: 22g

• Protein: 3.8g

• Sugar: 44g

• Cholesterol: 24mg

Roasted Pears

• Servings: 4 • Preparation time: 10 minutes • Cook time: 20 minutes •

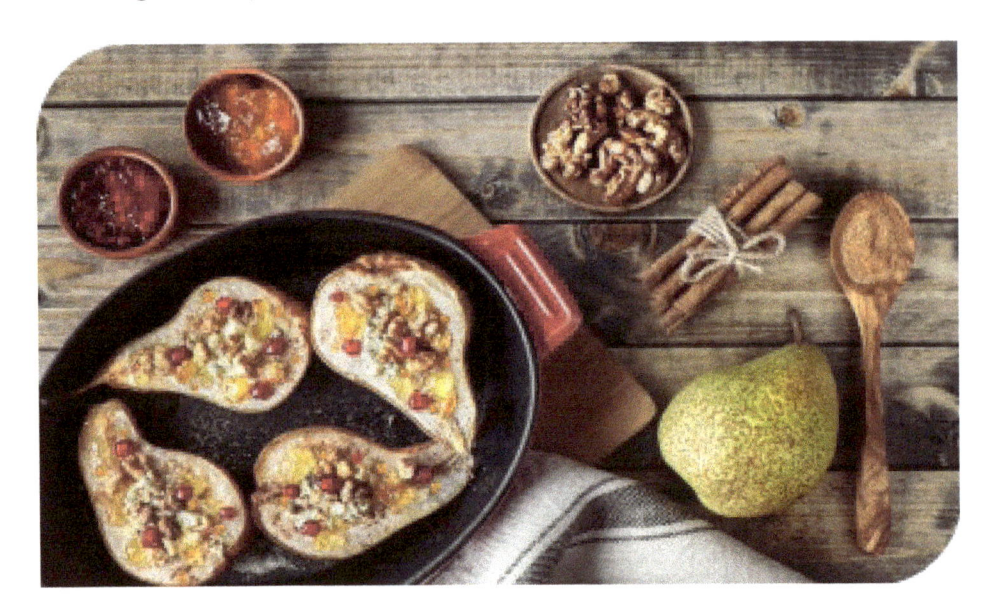

TASTY

Ingredients

- 4 pears in shell, well washed
- 50 g raisins
- 2 tablespoons sugar-free jam the one you like the most
- 1 teaspoon honey
- 1 pinch cinnamon powder

Steps to Cook

1. Wash the pears, hollowed out by removing the core.
2. Separate the pulp.
3. Mix the chosen jam with the pulp of the pears, honey and raisins and cinnamon.
4. Fill the pears with that mixture.
5. Place the pears in the fryer.
6. In the container place a glass of water.
7. Cook for 20 minutes at 1800C.
8. Serve them alone or accompanied with a scoop of vanilla ice cream.

Nutritional Information

- Calories: 84
- Carbohydrates: 22g
- Fat: 1g
- Protein: 1g
- Sugar: 35g
- Cholesterol: 300mg

Gluten Free Yogurt Cupcake

• Servings: 3 • Preparation time: 3 minutes • Cook time: 40 minutes •

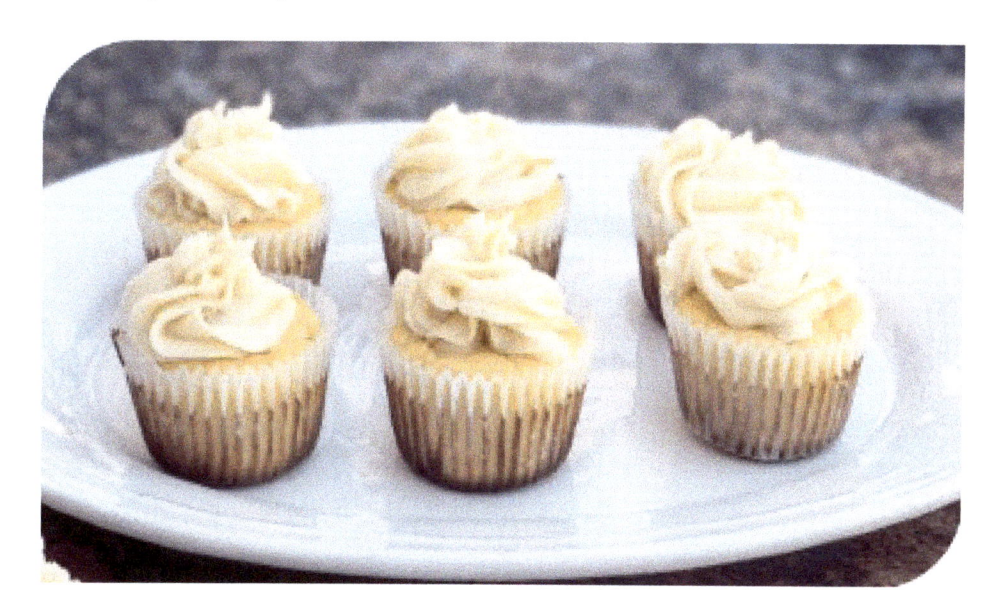

CREAMY

Ingredients

- 1 Greek yogurt
- 3 eggs
- 4 ½ oz. sugar
- 3 oz. cream
- 1 ½ oz. sunflower oil
- 1 ½ oz. butter
- 6 oz. gluten-free flour
- Salt
- 1 sachet yeast

Steps to Cook

1. Put the eggs, yogurt and sugar in the air fryer. Mix well. Add the rest of the ingredients and mix.

2. Put the dough in the cake container, previously brushed with oil. Preheat the fryer and put the mold with the dough for 40 minutes at 170ºC.

3. When it cools, we unmold and decorate to taste.

Nutritional Information

- Calories: 131
- Carbohydrates: 16g
- Fat: 6.3g
- Protein: 2.4g
- Sugar: 0.5g
- Cholesterol: 33.7mg

Tatin Mini Cake

• Servings:6 • Preparation time: 10 minutes • Cook time: 30 minutes •

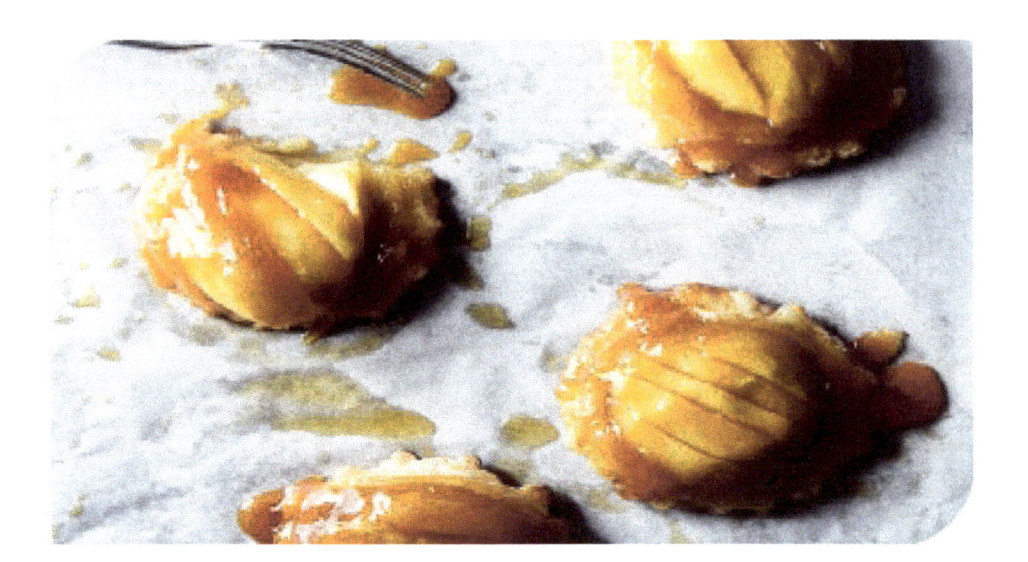

SPONGY

Ingredients

- 3 ½ oz. flour
- 1 ½ oz. cold butter
- 5 tsp water
- 1 pinch of salt
- 1 apple
- Lemon juice
- 1 oz. sugar
- ½ oz. butter

Steps to Cook

1. Put the salt in the flour and the cold butter. Mix everything until it is like sand. Add the 5 tsp of water and mix until obtaining a homogeneous mass. Wrap it in transparent paper and reserve. In a clay pot put the sugar and butter and let it melt and toast. Peel the apple, use the lemon juice to spread it. When your sugar and butter are already browned, put the apples on top, and place them tightly, cover the entire surface very well. Leave the apples caramelizing for 15 to 20 minutes; control them.

2. While, stretch the dough. You can do it as you find it easier. Once the apples are caramelized, top with the short crust pastry. Cut what is left and adjust to the contour.

3. Preheat the fryer to 160ºC, and put the cake for about 15 minutes.

Nutritional Information

- Calories: 355.7
- Carbohydrates: 62.9g
- Fat: 12.3g
- Protein: 2.1g
- Sugar: 25g
- Cholesterol: 30.7mg

Rabas

• Servings: 2 • Preparation time: 5 minutes • Cook time: 10 minutes •

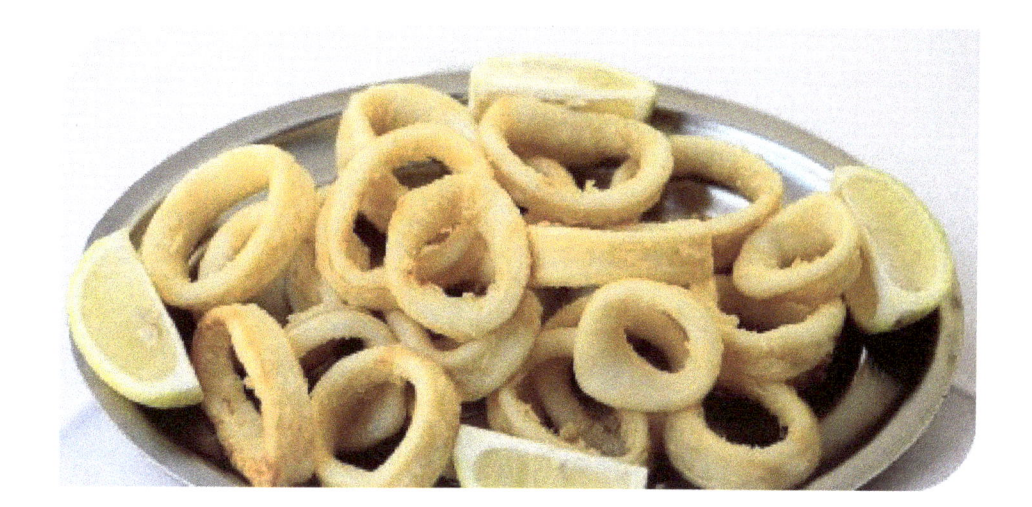

CRUNCHY

Ingredients

- 16 rabas
- 1 egg
- Bread crumbs
- Condiments: salt, pepper, sweet paprika

Steps to Cook

1. If they are frozen put them in hot water and they boil for 2 minutes.

2. Remove and dry well.

3. Beat the egg and season to taste, salt, pepper and sweet paprika. Place in the egg.

4. Bread with breadcrumbs. Place on sticks.

5. Place in the fryer for 5 minutes at 160ºC. Remove

9. Sprinkle with fritolin and place 5 more minutes at 200ºC.

Nutritional Information

- Calories: 200
- Carbohydrates: 1g
- Fat: 1g
- Protein: 1g
- Sugar: 0g
- Cholesterol: 0mg

Conclusion

Enjoying a delicious and healthy food that is oil-free is much easier if you do it with an oil-free fryer since these are the only fryers on the domestic market that offer us to enjoy any food, whether fried or not, without that it is necessary to use a large amount of oil, making the dishes much simpler to prepare and, above all, healthier.

The cooking time of oil-free fryers is somewhat longer than with traditional fryers. The most comfortable thing is that you review the instruction book of your fryer without oil and look at the recommended cooking times for each type of food, since depending on the food and the type of cooking you choose, the times will vary.

However, despite the extra cooking time, it is worth waiting a bit to eat a delicious and healthy version of your favorite dish. In the same way, it should be mentioned that the oil-free fries that can be obtained with this type of fryers offer a clear advantage that is that in addition to having a healthier diet, it is possible to avoid the unpleasant sensation that food usually leaves full of fat.

The capacity of oil-free deep fryers varies from one liter of capacity to 5 liters, and with anyone you can cook practically any type of food either at the same time or during several batches. And through its timer and control system, you can keep the temperature under control, as well as the time it takes for the oil-free deep fryer to prepare food more healthily.

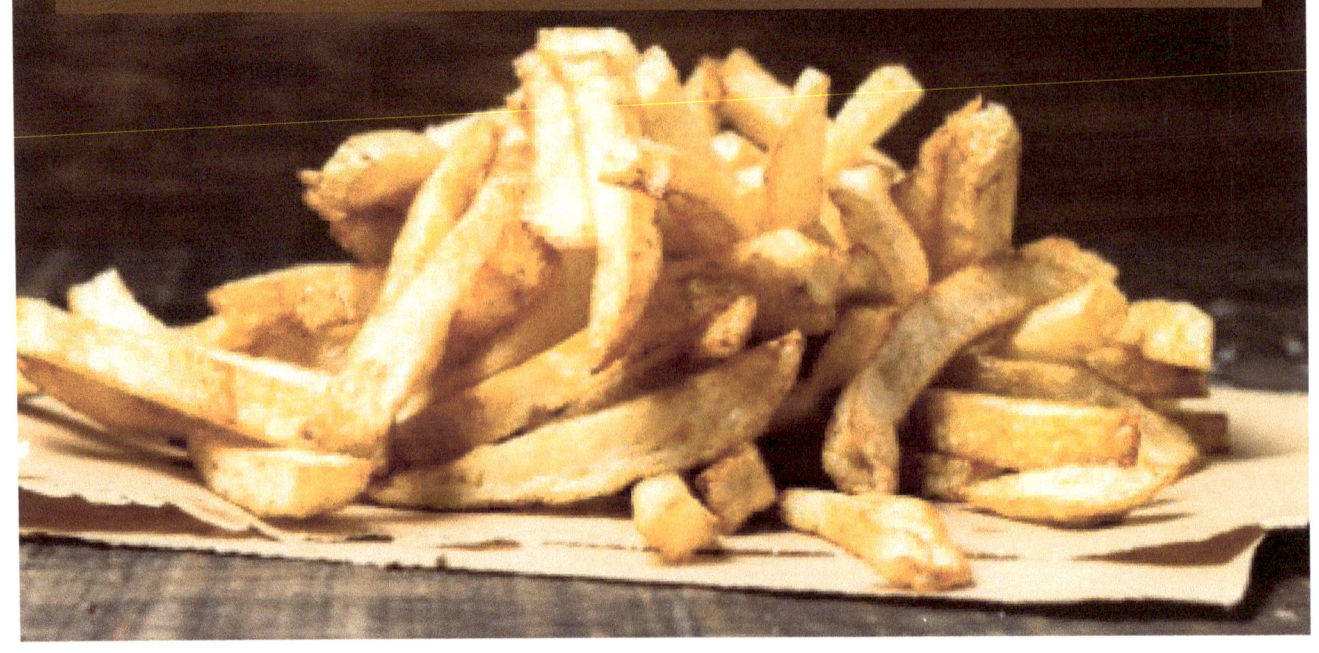

Lightning Source UK Ltd.
Milton Keynes UK
UKHW051334211020
371897UK00002B/58